RHEUMATOLOGY
G U I D E B O O K

D0784544

RHEUMATOLOGY
G U I D E B O O K
A Step-by-Step Guide to Diagnosis and Treatment

R. Ferrari
University of Alberta, Edmonton, Alberta, Canada

J. Cash
Cleveland Clinic Foundation, Cleveland, Ohio, USA

P. Maddison
Royal National Hospital for Rheumatic Diseases, Bath, UK

βIOS
SCIENTIFIC
PUBLISHERS

© **BIOS Scientific Publishers Limited, 1996**

First published 1996

A CIP catalogue record for this book is available from the British Library.

ISBN 1 859962 15 7

BIOS Scientific Publishers Ltd
9 Newtec Place, Magdalen Road, Oxford OX4 1RE, UK.
Tel. +44 (0)1865 726286. Fax +44 (0)1865 246823
World Wide Web home page: http://www.Bookshop.co.uk/BIOS/

This book is dedicated to the memory of
Giovanni Russo, William Henry Wright, Iris Vaughan
and Nikki Brenda Dawn Dœrksen.

Important Note from the Publisher

The information contained within this book was obtained by BIOS Scientific Publishers Ltd from sources believed by us to be reliable. However, while every effort has been made to ensure its accuracy, no responsiblity for loss or injury whatsoever occasioned to any person acting or refraining from action as a result of information contained herein can be accepted by the authors or publishers.

The reader should remember that medicine is a constantly evolving science and while the authors and publishers have ensured that all dosages, applications and practices are based on current indications, there may be specific practices which differ between communities. You should always follow the guidelines laid down by the manufacturers of specific products and the relevant authorities in the country in which you are practising.

Typeset by Florencetype Ltd, Stoodleigh, Tiverton, Devon, UK.
Printed by Redwood Books, Trowbridge, UK.

Contents

Section 4
Localized pain and swelling 99

Section 5
Outside the algorithm 145

Section 6
Treatment 193

Appendix 1
Physiotherapy exercises   **209**

Appendix 2
Soft-tissue inflammatory disorders (including shoulder arthritis)   **221**

Appendix 3
Joint aspiration and injection techniques   **223**

Further reading   **229**

Index   **231**

THE ALGORITHM

DIFFUSE PAIN

DIFFUSE PAIN
Chronic pain syndromes
Polymyalgia rheumatica
Malignancy

JOINT PAIN AND/OR STIFFNESS

LOCALIZED PAIN

LOCALIZED PAIN NEAR OR AT JOINT

NO JOINT SWELLING
Osteoarthritis
Tendinitis/Bursitis
Systemic lupus erythematosus

LOCALIZED PAIN + SWELLING

OBJECTIVE JOINT SWELLING

Mono-articular
Brief episode(s) (days)
  Palindromic arthritis
  Crystal arthropathy
  Septic arthritis
Chronic or prolonged episodes
  Crystal arthropathy
  Spondyloarthropathy

Polyarticular
Rheumatoid arthritis
Systemic lupus erythematosus
Spondyloarthropathy
Crystal arthropathy

Abbreviations

5-ASA	5-acetylsalicylic acid
ACR	American College of Rheumatology
AIDS	acquired immunodeficiency syndrome
ANA	anti-nuclear antibodies
ANCA	anti-neutrophil cytoplasmic antibodies
anti-dsDNA	antibodies to double stranded deoxyribonucleic acid
anti-Jo-1	antibodies to histidyl-transfer ribonucleic acid synthetase antigen
anti-La/SSB	antibody to RNA protein antigen
anti-PM-1	antibodies to nucleolar protein complex antigen
anti-RNP	antibodies to ribonucleoprotein
anti-Ro/SSA	antibody to RNA protein particle antigen
anti-Scl-70	antibodies to topoisomerase antigen
anti-Sm	antibodies to Smith antigen
ARA	American Rheumatism Association
ASA	acetylsalicylic acid
AZT	azidothymidine (zidovudine)
bid	Latin *bis in die* – twice a day
c-ANCA	diffuse cytoplasmic staining anti-neutrophil cytoplasmic antibodies
C1	first cervical vertebral level
C2	second cervical vertebral level
C5	fifth cervical vertebral level
CBC	complete blood count
CK	creatine kinase
cm	centimeter
CNS	central nervous system
COPD	chronic obstructive pulmonary disease
CREST	Calcinosis, Raynaud's phenomenon, Esophageal hypomotility, Sclerodactyly, Telangiectasia
CT	computed tomography
dL	deciliter
DIP	distal interphalangeal
DISH	diffuse idiopathic skeletal hyperostosis
dsDNA	double stranded deoxyribonucleic acid
EMG	electromyography

ESR	erythrocyte sedimentation rate
GI	gastrointestinal
H$_2$-blocker	histamine-2 receptor blocker
HIV	human immunodeficiency virus
HLA-B27	histocompatability antigen B27
IM	intramuscular
INR	international normalized ratio
IP	interphalangeal
IV	intravenous
L1-L4	from first to fourth lumbar vertebral levels
L3	third lumbar vertebral level
L3-L4	from third to fourth lumbar vertebral levels
L4	fourth lumbar vertebral level
LDH	lactate dehydrogenase
LE	lupus erythematosus
MCP	metacarpophalangeal
MCTD	mixed connective tissue disease
MRI	magnetic resonance imaging
MTP	metatarsophalangeal
N	normal
NSAIDs	nonsteroidal anti-inflammatory drugs
p-ANCA	perinuclear staining anti-neutrophil cytoplasmic antibodies
Pap	Papanicolaou
PIP	proximal interphalangeal
po	*per os* (by mouth)
prn	Latin *pro re nata* – according as circumstances may require
PSS	progressive systemic sclerosis
PT	prothrombin time
PTT	partial thromboplastin time
q4h	every 4 hours
q6h	every 6 hours
q8h	every 8 hours
q12h	every 12 hours
q24h	every 24 hours
qd	Latin *quaque die* – every day
qhs	Latin *quaque hora somni* – every bedtime
qid	Latin *quater in die* – four times a day
RA	rheumatoid arthritis
RF	rheumatoid factor
RNA	ribonucleic acid
sc	subcutaneous
SGOT	serum glutamic-oxaloacetic transaminase
SLE	systemic lupus erythematosus
T6-T9	from sixth to ninth thoracic vertebral levels
T8	eighth thoracic vertebral level

TB	tuberculosis
TENS	transcutaneous electrical nerve stimulation
TIA	transient ischemic attack
tid	Latin *ter in die* – three times a day
tid-qid	from three to four times a day
TMJ	temporomandibular joint
TSH	thyroid stimulating hormone
VDRL	venereal disease research laboratory syphilis test
WBC	white blood cell

Preface

Rheumatology Guidebook is designed to simplify the assessment and management of the patient with a rheumatic complaint, providing the practical concepts which rheumatologists use every day. Many of these practical aspects are not available in the rheumatology literature, even though rheumatologists rely on them immensely.

It is the lack of these essential concepts that makes rheumatology apparently difficult for nonrheumatologists, yet the concepts, once explained, and then applied, make most rheumatic diseases easily assessed and managed by any physician.

Rheumatology Guidebook first deals with the use of an algorithm that reflects, in part, the process rheumatologists go through in order to make a diagnosis, using the answers to specific initial questions to reach a distinct number of diagnostic possibilities. This algorithmic approach is combined with an understanding of serology and the diagnostic criteria for rheumatoid arthritis, systemic lupus erythematosus, and spondyloarthropathies. What the serologic tests are for, how they should be interpreted, and when to order (or not to order) them is discussed. It is then demonstrated how to use the history, physical examination and laboratory tests in pursuing the diagnostic criteria.

The chapters proceed through the algorithm as you would encounter a patient whose complaint brings you to a certain part of the algorithm. As each specific disease is discussed, there is a reiteration of the way in which the information in the previous chapters should be used. Diagnosis is emphasised, followed by management. Where appropriate, case scenarios are used to illustrate decision-making in certain commonly encountered situations. DOs and DON'Ts are provided as a further guide to decision-making. Later chapters deal with the practical aspects of therapy, both drugs and physiotherapy.

This text would not have been possible without the suggestions and critique of others in its production, special thanks to the rheumatologists of the University of Alberta for their instruction and advice.

R. Ferrari, J. Cash and P. Maddison

Section 1 – Introduction

Approach to rheumatic complaints

The practice of rheumatology is not difficult. The most important diagnostic test is a precise medical history. This is followed up by a careful physical examination of the area(s) involved, which frequently confirms the diagnosis. Ordering investigations blindly, when rheumatic disease is not apparent clinically, is unwise. Such investigations merely add to costs, delay the diagnosis, and lead to inappropriate referrals for diseases that the patient does not have. Throughout this book, note how specific aspects of the history and examination alone make the diagnosis. In most referrals, rheumatologists do little but ask the right questions. Anyone can learn this skill.

How does one get from the patient's symptoms to the diagnosis? First, understand how patients with rheumatic diseases express their symptoms, and how rheumatologists inquire about those symptoms. There are many examples where careful questioning prevents misconceptions.

Stiffness, for example, is a common complaint. Some patients actually mean 'sore' when they say 'stiff', because they cannot move their fingers due to pain (hence their fingers must be stiff). Ask the patient about their stiffness. Patients with true stiffness realize that if they move their joints they can get rid of the stiffness, even though the pain has not resolved and they are still 'sore'. Important stiffness is usually of greater than one hour duration. Shorter periods of stiffness are common in osteoarthritis, tendinitis, and fibromyalgia. Patients with prominent inflammatory conditions, such as rheumatoid arthritis, ankylosing spondylitis, or polymyalgia rheumatica will have their most marked stiffness in the morning, because most of their joints and muscles have been at rest for several hours. Patients with noninflammatory, or mild local inflammatory conditions (tendinitis) will have stiffness at various times of the day, waxing and waning, often worst in the evenings.

Another example of more careful assessment of the patient is concerned with joint swelling. When a patient complains of joint swelling, they should be asked to contact a physician when it occurs, so that it can be documented objectively. Even if the patient says they can no longer 'wear their rings on the fingers', swelling is not proven. Remember that when arthritis does produce swelling it is very obvious. If the physician has to look extremely close for subtle differences or changes and can see a few millimetres difference when comparing a

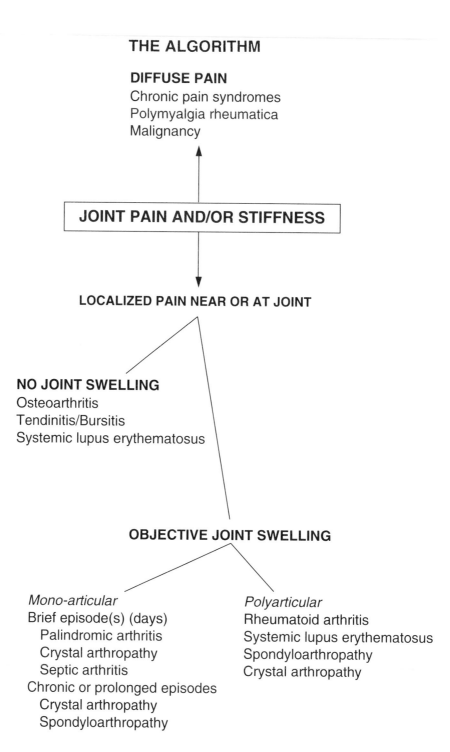

THE ALGORITHM

DIFFUSE PAIN
Chronic pain syndromes
Polymyalgia rheumatica
Malignancy

JOINT PAIN AND/OR STIFFNESS

LOCALIZED PAIN NEAR OR AT JOINT

NO JOINT SWELLING
Osteoarthritis
Tendinitis/Bursitis
Systemic lupus erythematosus

OBJECTIVE JOINT SWELLING

Mono-articular
Brief episode(s) (days)
  Palindromic arthritis
  Crystal arthropathy
  Septic arthritis
Chronic or prolonged episodes
  Crystal arthropathy
  Spondyloarthropathy

Polyarticular
Rheumatoid arthritis
Systemic lupus erythematosus
Spondyloarthropathy
Crystal arthropathy

DIFFUSE PAIN

LOCALIZED PAIN

LOCALIZED PAIN + SWELLING

Fig. 1.1 Algorithm.

'swollen' joint with a normal one, the chances are no swelling exists. The patient may believe it exists, and this is accepted as a real symptom of certain illnesses such as fibromyalgia and other chronic pain syndromes. Whether or not the physician can objectively find swelling makes a significant difference to diagnosis. Too often patients are told they have arthritis when they actually have fibromyalgia; one condition has objective swelling, the other does not. A patient only has swelling when that swelling has been observed.

Rheumatologists must also make note of the way certain patients describe their symptoms. When a patient complains of pain around the joints and spine, and describes it 'as if I had been shot', or 'as if my muscle was tearing in two', then most likely they have a chronic pain syndrome.

Using a series of careful questions, an algorithmic approach may be adopted (*Figure 1.1*). This algorithm is useful in practice, and forms a template for the organization of this book. The upper part of the algorithm refers to those disorders in which the patient, upon careful questioning, is found to have diffuse pain. The book deals with these disorders first. The middle part of the algorithm includes those disorders with localized pain but no swelling, and the lower part of the algorithm considers localized pain and swelling, either monoarticular or polyarticular. The text will consider these two parts of the algorithm in turn. Finally, there are a number of rheumatic diseases which are not shown in the algorithm, chiefly because they do not typically present with joint pain or stiffness. These sections will deal with back pain, neck pain, scleroderma, polymyositis, vasculitis, osteoporosis, and reflex sympathetic dystrophy. One can sometimes be alerted to these disorders by specific presenting complaints. Thus, some of these sections will be introduced with 'When a patient has x, consider y'.

The following section explains exactly how the algorithmic approach is used in practice, emphasizing the need to ask the right questions.

Section 1 – Introduction

Asking the right
questions

The path to a correct diagnosis begins with the right questions. That is, rheumatologists, perhaps more often than in any other discipline of medicine, rely on patterns of symptom expression as the key clues to the diagnosis. They elicit these patterns by carefully chosen questions. Because so many rheumatic diseases are diagnosed on the basis of history and physical examination (and in some cases the history suffices), failure to ask the right questions inevitably keeps the physician from arriving at the correct diagnosis.

In addition, some patients make their own diagnoses and expect the physician to just confirm them. It is worthwhile to discourage patients from using medical terms or relaying the diagnosis of previous physicians. These statements frequently bias the physician and prevent the patient from actually defining their symptoms.

Patients do not have an appreciation of the anatomic and pathophysiologic correlation to symptom expression in rheumatic diseases. Physicians may be led astray when the patient tells them they have pain in their hands because they accept that statement, and proceed with the assumption that the patient has defined their pattern of pain correctly; often they have not.

It is always important to ask about and document the chronology of the symptoms or illness. The duration and pattern of symptoms is often important in the diagnosis of many rheumatic diseases, as will become apparent later.

The first question in the algorithm: 'Where exactly are your symptoms?' decides whether or not one takes the threatening, winding, and complex path to a multitude of diseases and need for investigations (the lower sections of the algorithm), or the gentle stroll to the chronic pain syndromes which require no investigations, and no medications, but merely a long talk.

Consider a patient who complains of hand arthritis:

Doctor   Where is your pain?
Patient   In my hands.
Doctor   Please point to the sites exactly. Which parts of the hand are involved?

Patient demonstrates that the whole of both hands are involved.

Doctor	Does the pain go anywhere else from your hands?
Patient	Sometimes it gets into my arms and up to my shoulders.
Doctor	What about your neck?
Patient	Oh, yes, sometimes from my neck right down, but it's my hands that are the worst.
Doctor	Tell me, aside from your whole arm pain, do you have any other aches and pains?
Patient	Oh yes, but I am here for my hand arthritis.
Doctor	What about your knees, hips, and legs in general?
Patient	Oh yes, especially here and here and here.
Doctor	Are there times when you ache all over.
Patient	Oh yes, you wouldn't believe it.

If the doctor had taken the patient's complaint of hand arthritis and not bothered to ask about the localization of pain, then he or she would have immediately strayed down the path towards tendinitis, bursitis, arthritis, and systemic lupus erythematosus (SLE): a mistake, and a disfavor to the patient, because that would mean leaving the patient with the idea that they may have some terrible form of arthritis, need lots of investigations, and maybe referral to a rheumatologist.

Instead, however, with the information that is gained by defining the pattern of diffuse versus focal localization of pain (Where exactly are your symptoms?), the correct path has been chosen, and the patient must have one of either a chronic pain syndrome, polymyalgia rheumatica (if the patient is over 55 years of age and has an elevated erythrocyte sedimentation rate (ESR)), or in the elderly, a malignancy (in which risk factors are present, tender points are not prominent, and anorexia and weight loss are often present). Chronic pain syndromes and polymyalgia rheumatica are dealt with on pages 26 and 39. There, more questions are given to ask the patient and confirm the diagnosis. The patient's symptom of hand pain has now led to a few distinct possibilities, simply because the right questions were asked. The diagnosis has not been made until proceeding to the questions for the two diagnostic considerations, but the task has been made much easier.

Some may argue that a patient who has a chronic pain syndrome such as fibromyalgia may develop true tendinitis or bursitis, which is missed because every complaint they bring is going to occur in a setting of chronic diffuse pain. Although some physicians claim they are able to distinguish tendinitis in a patient with chronic whole arm pain, most will find this difficult.

To miss tendinitis in a patient with whole arm pain, however, may not be a tragedy. It is unlikely that specific therapy for tendinitis would alter their symptoms overall. Equally, if the patient with whole arm pain happens to have osteoarthritis of the hands, it may not be a great loss to fail to detect it. This type of hand arthritis has an excellent prognosis, and is far less limiting (as far as the patient is concerned) than the whole arm pain. Further, a patient with whole arm pain has probably tried nonsteroidal anti-inflammatory drugs (NSAIDs) or acetaminophen (paracetamol), which could be used to treat osteoarthritis, and yet they will say they are not much better for having done so. The same is often true for local treatment modalities. So the management, and the overall outcome for the patient with whole arm pain and osteoarthritis of the hands may not be any different for having identified both problems.

It may not seem ideal that one may miss some minor condition in a patient with a chronic pain syndrome, but there is far greater harm bestowed upon patients in the reverse scenario: if they have fibromyalgia, but are told they have tendinitis or arthritis. The general public often connotes the word 'arthritis' with life-long disability, and a prognosis that includes crippling pain. Letting a patient with fibromyalgia have the misdiagnosis of arthritis can be disastrous.

The cases below further illustrate how a few key initial questions narrow the diagnostic possibilities. (Remember that in addition to the questions set out in the algorithm, it is important to document the chronology of the symptoms.)

Consider a patient who has pain in the shoulder:

Doctor	Where is your pain?
Patient	It is right in my shoulder sometimes, with some pain in my upper arm, and in the back of my shoulder.
Doctor	Does the pain go anywhere else?
Patient	No.
Doctor	What about your neck?
Patient	No.
Doctor	Aside from your shoulder pain, do you have aches and pains elsewhere?
Patient	I get a sore back from time to time, but that's about it.
Doctor	What about your hands, hips, knees?
Patient	No problems there.

Now one is travelling down the algorithm because the patient has localized their pain to one region. Swelling in the shoulder joint is rare, except in cases of septic arthritis or pseudogout, whereby a patient will have so much shoulder pain that they (and the physician) cannot move their shoulder much. The patient needs a joint aspiration if one suspects septic arthritis or pseudogout. In the absence of swelling the choices on the algorithm include: tendinitis/bursitis; osteoarthritis; and systemic lupus erythematosus (SLE).

Proceed now to page 42 on the painful shoulder, and the diagnosis will be confirmed by the examination technique described. Shoulder pain is not a presentation of SLE, but even if it was, the information presented in the following topic on diagnostic criteria (page 10) would make it simple for one to discard this possibility. Once again, a symptom has been reduced to a few distinct possibilities by asking certain questions.

Now consider a patient with painful feet:

Doctor	Where is your pain?
Patient	Under the balls of my feet and sometimes across the top and over my shins.

Doctor	Does the pain go anywhere else?
Patient	No.
Doctor	Aside from your feet, do you have aches and pains elsewhere?
Patient	No.
Doctor	What about your hands, hips, knees, back and neck?
Patient	No.

Again the patient has localized their pain to one body part, and so one is travelling down the algorithm. The patient does not report swelling and none is found. Thus the patient must have one of: tendinitis/bursitis; osteoarthritis; or SLE.

Again, one can go through the questions of SLE if you wish, and one will be left with tendinitis/bursitis or osteoarthritis. If one proceeds to the topic on the painful foot or ankle (page 83), the examination will give the diagnosis, and allow one to choose between the diagnostic possibilities. This patient happens to have collapsed arches. Diagnosis made. No further investigation needed.

Next, consider a patient complaining of hand arthritis, but in whom joint swelling is documented:

Doctor	Where is your pain?
Patient	In my hands.
Doctor	Show me exactly.

(Patient shows that pain is in metacarpophalangeal (MCP) joints and wrists of both hands.)

Doctor	What about the other joints?
Patient	They seem fine.
Doctor	Do you have any other aches and pains?
Patient	No.

You now examine the hands and there is swelling. (If there is not on this occasion, but the patient said there was, one needs to make an arrangement to see that patient the next time they have swelling.) The diagnosis of arthritis in these hands is straightforward. The patient has localized pain and swelling is documented. Therefore one has moved down the algorithm, with the next question being 'How many joints?' There is more than one joint involved so one of the following must be considered: rheumatoid arthritis; SLE; spondyloarthropathy; or crystal arthropathy

Now go to the diagnostic criteria for the first three (see the topic diagnostic criteria, page 10), ask about historical criteria, examine for the physical criteria, and perform the laboratory tests listed. (One does not have to do the tests for spondyloarthropathy unless the patient has the clinical features.) Combine this with joint aspiration to look for crystals and you will have a diagnosis. The details of this process will become clearer as the book proceeds, but the key concept is that three initial questions ('Where is your pain?', 'Is there objective swelling?', and 'How many joints are involved?') led to these four diagnostic possibilities. The remaining process of diagnosis is simply another set of specific questions to be answered.

Finally, consider a patient who develops episodic swelling in the knee:

Doctor   Where is your pain?
Patient   When it happens, in my right knee only.
Doctor   Any other joints involved or other aches and pains?
Patient   No.

One is again moving down the algorithm and the patient has come today because the last time they came, the attack was gone. There is only one joint involved, and so the patient must have one of: palindromic arthritis; septic arthritis; or crystal arthropathy. Osteoarthritis of the knee can produce episodic swelling as well, although some of these episodes may actually be crystal-induced. (See page 92 on osteoarthritis.)

Read the topics palindromic arthritis, septic arthritis, and crystal arthropathy (pages 100, 113 and 102 respectively).

The patient is having brief, episodic attacks, so they cannot have septic arthritis. If this was the first episode, however, one would have to rule out septic arthritis. In this case, however, the two possibilities remaining are palindromic arthritis and crystal arthropathy. Aspirate the joint (or send the patient to someone who will) and with knowledge of palindromic arthritis one will be able to give this patient a diagnosis. Again, by asking three initial questions ('Where is your pain?', 'Is there objective swelling?', and 'How many joints are involved?'), the diagnostic possibilities have been narrowed and are then easily discerned when one considers what is discussed in the topics on those possibilities.

One might argue that in some cases such a methodical approach will fail if there is an unusual presentation of the disease, and that such an approach is overly simplistic. This is true, but such unusual cases are rare. Rheumatologists' offices are not filled with unusual cases. They are filled with straightforward, misdiagnosed cases, that could have been avoided by the use of the algorithm; that is, by asking the right questions.

Discussion of the following topics will start with the symptom, and proceed as if one has used the algorithm to place the patient's diagnosis within a limited number of distinct possibilities.

First, we will proceed up the algorithm, that is, chronic pain syndromes and polymyalgia rheumatica, as if the patient has presented with diffuse pain. Then we will proceed down the algorithm (the patient has complained of well-localized pain and no swelling) to discuss tendinitis/bursitis and osteoarthritis as diagnoses of regional pain (and SLE later). Finally, we will discuss those diseases which present with the patient having both localized pain and swelling: the remainder of the algorithm. Some other diseases are not included in the algorithm, being far less prevalent, and diagnosed by a different approach. These diseases will be introduced in their respective topics with a statement like 'When a patient presents with this symptom or sign think x', so that one will have a stark reminder of when the patient's diagnosis is outside the above algorithm. Before all of this, however, it is necessary to understand the diagnostic criteria and serology used by rheumatologists.

Section 1 – Introduction

Diagnostic criteria

Diagnostic criteria were designed by the American Rheumatism Association (ARA), the American College of Rheumatology (ACR), and others to maintain uniformity of patient inclusion into clinical or epidemiologic studies (see *Tables 1.1–1.8*). The criteria primarily emphasized facets of the disease that distinguish that disease from alternative rheumatic disease diagnoses. One must realize, however, that these criteria do not entirely define the clinical presentation or many of the important manifestations of the various diseases. Patients should be asked about symptoms that, even though they are not diagnostic criteria, are important in treatment decisions (e.g. Raynaud's phenomenon).

Rheumatologists who have had many years of experience, who have seen the widest spectrum of each of these diseases, and who have observed how the natural history of each presentation evolves, can make a diagnosis without necessarily meeting diagnostic criteria. A rheumatologist would be able to defend that diagnosis on the basis of clinical experience. For most other physicians, however, this is not the case and the diagnostic criteria offer a means by which one can have confidence in making or ruling out a diagnosis, and by which to defend that diagnosis. As well, the diagnostic criteria remind us of which symptoms or signs of diseases are the most important in diagnosis. Indeed, the diagnostic criteria are a particularly useful framework from which the clinician can assess a patient with suspected SLE. Patients with SLE may have fatigue, weight loss, fever, and a number of symptoms, but the most important diagnostic symptoms and signs to be sought lie in the diagnostic criteria. Without inquiring about these, the diagnostic process is not advanced much further. Finally, the diagnostic criteria are helpful in telling the physician when serology is indicated. If a patient has none or just one of the diagnostic criteria, ordering serology is not useful, because even if positive, there would not be enough reason to make the diagnosis. As patients begin to accumulate diagnostic criteria, however, such as three criteria for SLE or for rheumatoid arthritis, positive serology will allow the diagnosis to be confirmed.

An example of the utility of diagnostic criteria can be found in the common clinical scenario, for instance, of deciding whether or not a patient with a positive anti-nuclear antibody (ANA) assay (see page 20) and arthritis has SLE. Although most patients with SLE are ANA positive, the finding of this and arthritis is not specific enough for only SLE, and does not satisfy the diagnostic criteria for SLE. Does this patient have SLE? No; the criteria as described below are not met. This diagnosis (or misdiagnosis) of SLE obviously has important treatment, prognostic, and psychosocial implications for the patient.

Finally, one must realize that systemic rheumatic diseases are not static. They are fluid. It is not unusual for diseases (or patients with three criteria) to evolve over a period of years, so that a clear diagnosis is defined. (Do not confuse this, however, with believing that a patient who meets only one criterion for SLE, and yet has plenty of symptoms, is going to develop SLE.) Because of the evolution of rheumatic diseases, these criteria should be kept in mind each time the patient is seen. Until a firm diagnosis can be made, symptomatic treatment (e.g. NSAIDs) is used with periodic re-evaluation of the patient for diagnostic criteria.

As another example of using the diagnostic criteria for SLE, consider the patient with this complaint:

'I wonder if I have lupus, doctor. Do I?'

One may ask the patient about the localization of their pain and would find it is diffuse. The algorithmic approach takes one up the algorithm in this case, and one would begin asking questions from the topic on chronic pain syndromes and polymyalgia rheumatica (pages 26 and 39, respectively). SLE is not on that part of the algorithm, but if one wanted to reassure the patient, one could, knowing the diagnostic criteria for SLE, proceed as follows:

First, no serology!

Doctor	Have you had any rashes on your face?
Patient	I sometimes get very itchy, and my face gets swollen, with pain in my jaws, but no rash.
Doctor	Does sunlight cause a rash, or are you allergic to the sun?
Patient	No.
Doctor	Do you experience joint pain or swelling?
Patient	Yes. I have had pain in pretty much all my joints, and I can't get my rings off any more.
Doctor	Have you ever had a seizure?
Patient	No.
Doctor	Have you ever had chest pain? (If the patient says no, then move to next question, but if they say yes, they must have a documented history of pericarditis or pleuritis with pain on inspiration and usually hospital admission or at least a diagnosis in emergency of either of these. The pain of pericarditis or pleuritis does not go away in a couple of days either.)
Patient	Last week, I had this pain that went around my chest and up the back of my head.

(On examination, the doctor notes that no joint swelling exists, and notes a normal complete blood count (CBC) and urinalysis.)

Doctor	From the information you have given me, and from my examination, I can reassure you that you do not have lupus.
Patient	But what about the positive lupus test and my symptoms?

Doctor   The ANA test should not really be called a lupus test, because while most patients with lupus have a positive ANA, there are many people who also have a positive ANA without having lupus. While some of the symptoms you have are seen in lupus patients, these symptoms are not specific for lupus, and many other illnesses cause them. Your illness is called fibromyalgia.

This is but one example of how the diagnostic criteria can be helpful. Others will be revealed in later sections.

Table 1.1   ARA/ACR criteria for diagnosis of rheumatoid arthritis (last revised in 1987)

1.	[a]Morning stiffness > 1 h
2.	[a]Arthritis of at least three types of joints proximal interphalangeal (PIP), metacarpophalangeal (MCP), wrist, elbow, knee, ankle, metatarsophalangeal (MTP)
3.	[a]Arthritis of hand joints
4.	[a]Symmetrical arthritis
5.	Rheumatoid nodules
6.	Rheumatoid factor
7.	Joint erosions on X-ray of wrists and hands

Four criteria = rheumatoid arthritis.

[a] Must be present for > 6 weeks, since polyarthritis of shorter duration may not be due to rheumatoid arthritis, and may spontaneously resolve without a diagnosis.

Table 1.2   ARA criteria for diagnosis of SLE (last revised in 1982)

1.	Malar rash (fixed erythematous patches, raised or flat, sparing nasolabial folds)
2.	Discoid rash (erythematous papules or plaques on head and neck, with scaling, follicular keratosis, atrophic scarring, and depigmentation)
3.	Photosensitive rash
4.	Oral or nasopharyngeal ulcers (usually painless)
5.	Arthritis (nonerosive, more than two joints)
6.	Serositis (pleural, pericardial, or peritoneal)
7.	Renal disease otherwise unexplained (proteinuria > 0.5 g/day or casts)
8.	CNS disorder (seizures or psychosis) otherwise unexplained
9.	Hematologic disorder (autoimmune hemolytic anemia, [a]leukopenia < 4.0 x 10^9/l, [a]lymphopenia < 1.5 x 10^9/l, or [a]thrombocytopenia < 100 x 10^9/l)
10.	Serology (positive lupus erythematosus (LE) cell prep, anti-DNA antibody, anti-Sm antibody, or VDRL [b]
11.	Positive anti-nuclear antibody (ANA)

Four criteria = SLE. Can only use one of the skin manifestations and one of the hematologic manifestations.

[a] Observed on more than one occasion.

[b] Most do not use these tests, but rather simply check for positive ANA.

Table 1.3 Criteria for diagnosis of seronegative spondyloarthropathies (adapted from Amor, 1991). Reference: Calin A (1993) Spondyloarthropathy, undifferentiated Spondyloarthritis and overlap. In: *Oxford Textbook of Rheumatology* (eds Maddison P J, Isenberg D A, Woo P and Glass D N). Oxford University Press, Oxford, p.668.

1.	Nocturnal pain or morning stiffness of lumbar or dorsal spine
2.	Asymmetric oligoarthritis
3.	Alternating right and left gluteal pain
4.	'Sausage' digit (characteristic swelling of whole digit)
5.	Plantar fasciitis
6.	Iritis
7.	Recent (< 1 month) nongonococcal urethritis/cervicitis or diarrhea prior to arthritis
8.	One of psoriasis, balanitis, or inflammatory bowel disease
9.	Sacroiliitis on X-ray
10.	Positive family history or HLA-B27 positive[a]
11.	Dramatic improvement with NSAIDs

Six criteria = definite seronegative spondyloarthropathy, but suspect on 1 and 11 alone, or arthritis and 7 or 8 alone.

[a] Do not order HLA-B27 unless for research purposes. It neither makes nor rules out the diagnosis of a spondyloarthropathy.

Note that these criteria remind one of the different types of spondyloarthropathy, that is, ankylosing spondylitis, reactive arthritis, psoriatic arthritis, and bowel-associated arthritis.

The remaining diagnostic criteria are less often used rigorously for the respective disorders.

Table 1.4 ARA criteria for diagnosis of systemic sclerosis

1.	Major criterion: proximal scleroderma (extends proximal to MCP joints)
2.	Minor criteria: sclerodactyly, pitting scars on fingertips, loss of distal finger pulp thickness, bibasilar lung crackles

One major and two minor criteria = systemic sclerosis

Table 1.5 Criteria for diagnosis of polymyositis/dermatomyositis (adapted from Bohan and Peter, 1975). Reference: Bohan A and Peter J B (1975) Polymyositis and dermatomyositis. *New Engl. J. Med.* **292**: 344–347.

1.	Progressive, symmetric proximal muscle weakness
2.	Muscle biopsy showing necrosis, phagocytosis, regeneration, inflammation
3.	Elevated creatinine kinase or aldolase
4.	Electromyography showing myopathic potentials, fibrillations, and complex repetitive discharges
5.	Rash of dermatomyositis (blue-red to violet papules on dorsum of hands, elbows, ankles, neck, and trunk – Gottron's papules)

All of 1–4 = polymyositis, all of 1–5 = dermatomyositis.

Table 1.6 Criteria for diagnosis of polymyalgia rheumatica (adapted from Jones and Hazleman, 1981). Reference: Jones J G and Hazleman B L (1981) The prognosis and management of polymyalgia rheumatica. *Annal. Int. Med.* **40**: 1–5.

1.	Shoulder and pelvic girdle muscular pain without true weakness
2.	Morning stiffness
3.	Duration of > 2 months
4.	Elevated ESR
5.	Normal creatinine kinase
6.	Absence of other inflammatory arthritis or malignancy
7.	Dramatic response to corticosteroids

All criteria required.

Table 1.7 ACR criteria for diagnosis for giant cell arteritis (1990). Reference: Dasgupta B, Panayi G S (1993) Polymyalgia rheumatica. In: *Oxford Textbook of Rheumatology* (eds Maddison P J, Isenberg D A, Woo P and Glass D N). Oxford University Press, Oxford, p. 866.

1.	Onset at age > 50 years
2.	New headache
3.	Temporal artery tenderness or reduced pulsation
4.	ESR > 50 mm/h
5.	Biopsy showing necrotizing arteritis (usually with multinucleated giant cells)

Three criteria = giant cell arteritis.

Table 1.8 ACR criteria for diagnosis of fibromyalgia (1990). Reference: Hazleman B (1993) Soft tissue rheumatism. In: *Oxford Textbook of Rheumatology* (eds Maddison P J, Isenberg D A, Woo P and Glass D N). Oxford University Press, Oxford, p. 946.

1.	History of diffuse > 2 months pain with all of the following: pain below and above waist pain on right and left upper trunk or low back pain
2.	Pain in 11 of 18 standard painful points on palpation suboccipital muscle insertions (2) low cervical C5–C7 (2) trapezius (2) supraspinatus origins (2) second costochondral junctions (2) lateral humeral epicondyles – 2 cm distal (2) gluteal (2) greater femoral trochanters (2) medial fat pads of knee (2)

DOs and DON'Ts of Diagnostic Criteria

DO consider using diagnostic criteria when trying to decide whether a patient has rheumatoid arthritis, SLE, or fibromyalgia and other chronic pain syndromes, etc. Realize that it may take time for one to be able to collect all the information needed to do so, but that the patient can be treated symptomatically while waiting.

DO feel confident in concluding that a patient does not have SLE if they meet too few of the diagnostic criteria.

DO feel confident in diagnosing a patient's aches and pains as a chronic pain syndrome when you have taken the appropriate history, examined for the appropriate physical findings, and have *clinically* ruled out other rheumatic diseases by the lack of specific findings.

DO realize that even rheumatologists sometimes cannot come up with a diagnosis even though a patient clearly has arthritis and other evidence of disease, and that a patient's arthritis can still be treated while awaiting for the diagnosis to become clear.

Obtaining a diagnosis

Combining the questions from the algorithm and the diagnostic criteria, one has a list of questions that if pursued in this fashion will lead to a diagnosis. Starting with 'Where is your pain?' the entire collection of questions is shown below (not all of them are needed, of course, when early questions lead to a diagnosis).

If diffuse pain: ask about symptoms and examine for signs (physical and laboratory) to be found in chronic pain syndromes, polymyalgia rheumatica, and malignancy.

If localized pain: objectively determine whether joint swelling is present or not.

If no swelling present: examine the region of pain to distinguish tendinitis/bursitis from osteoarthritis.

If swelling present: consider how many joints.

If more than one joint is involved at a given time: ask about and look for the diagnostic criteria listed for rheumatoid arthritis, SLE, spondyloarthropathy, and aspirate for crystal arthropathy.

Rheumatoid arthritis

Morning stiffness > 1 h?
Arthritis of at least three types of joint?
Arthritis of hand joints?
Symmetric involvement?
Rheumatoid nodules?
Rheumatoid factor positive?
Joint erosions on X-ray of wrists and hands?

Systemic lupus erythematosus

Malar rash? Discoid rash? Photosensitive rash?
Oral or nasopharyngeal ulcers?
Arthritis (nonerosive, more than two joints)?
Serositis (pleural, pericardial, or peritoneal)?
Renal disease otherwise unexplained (proteinuria > 0.5 g per day or casts)?
CNS disorder (seizures or psychosis) otherwise unexplained?

Hematologic disorder?
Positive ANA?

Spondyloarthropathy

Nocturnal pain or morning stiffness of lumbar or dorsal spine?
Asymmetric oligoarthritis?
Alternating right and left gluteal pain?
'Sausage' digit?
Plantar fasciitis?
Iritis?
Recent (< 1 month) nongonococcal urethritis/cervicitis or diarrhea?
One of psoriasis, balanitis, or inflammatory bowel disease?
Sacroiliitis on X-ray?
Dramatic improvement with NSAIDs?

Crystal arthropathy

Aspirate results?

If only one joint at a time: ask about symptoms in palindromic arthritis, ask about the diagnostic criteria for spondyloarthropathy, and aspirate for crystal arthropathy or septic arthritis.

Serology

There is no such thing as a 'collagen-vascular disease' screen. In general, one should never order a test for rheumatoid factor or anti-nuclear antibody (ANA) unless one has clear clinical and laboratory evidence otherwise of a rheumatic disease. Think about some of the diagnostic criteria listed on pages 10–14. If the patient lacks these, one should not order serology, because positive results will not take the diagnosis any further, but will only lead to confusion, worry, added expense, and inappropriate referrals.

Fatigue, shoulder ache, tennis elbow, numbness or tingling, arthritis in one joint, and spine disorders, with no other specific criteria present are not reasons for ordering serology. It must first be proven that there is actually a case of rheumatoid arthritis or the diagnostic criteria for SLE before ordering such tests.

Routine use of serology in patients lacking clinical evidence for a rheumatic disease will not increase the diagnostic yield. Instead, the physician is more often left with a false positive result for the disease in question, leading to inappropriate tests or referrals prompted by that false positive result. As shown on page 21, for example, a positive ANA test in a patient with right wrist pain does not allow for the diagnosis of SLE since more criteria than this must be met. As another example, the rheumatoid factor, although commonly seen in rheumatoid arthritis, is not specific for this disease, so that in a patient lacking other clinical criteria for the diagnosis of rheumatoid arthritis, a positive test is not useful. Further, some patients with rheumatoid arthritis lack the rheumatoid factor, yet can still receive the correct diagnosis, because there are other criteria met.

Erythrocyte sedimentation rate (ESR)

This is not a test for antibodies, but rather a reflection of an inflammatory process, and is commonly used (and abused) as such in patients presenting with rheumatic complaints. The best reasons for ordering an ESR are as follows.

Elderly patient with headache, sudden visual loss, diplopia, or jaw pain (giant cell arteritis).

Elderly patient with morning stiffness and pain in shoulder and hip girdle (polymyalgia rheumatica).

Following response to therapy in polymyositis, polymyalgia rheumatica, or rheumatoid arthritis.

The worst reasons for ordering an ESR are as follows.

When one has no idea of what is wrong with the patient (no help even if elevated, and not always reassuring if negative).

The patient clearly has signs of inflammation (redundant).

The upper limit of normal for the ESR is age and sex dependent. By the Westergren method, the upper limits can be calculated as follows:

For men: age divided by 2

For women: (age + 10) divided by 2.

So a 66-year-old woman may have an ESR that is normal up to (66 + 10) divided by 2 = 38.

The importance of knowing this range of normal is that many laboratories report a range of normal for patients under 25 years of age. It is therefore misleading when the result of 38, which is normal for a women of 66, is called abnormal by the laboratory.

This does not mean that an ESR under this upper limit excludes disease in a patient, and an abnormal ESR does not necessarily mean disease. (About 10% of patients with an unexplained elevated ESR will never be found to have a cause.)

Rheumatologists must therefore rely on the history and physical examination rather than the ESR. The worst mistake a physician can make is to order an ESR when not indicated, because this leads to unwarranted concerns.

Rheumatoid factor

This is not a 'rheumatoid arthritis' test. This test should be ordered when a patient has at least three other criteria for rheumatoid arthritis (see page 12), and one wants to add more strength to the diagnostic conclusion.

Rheumatoid factor is a misnomer since many patients who test positive for rheumatoid factor do not have rheumatoid arthritis. Rheumatoid factor can be detected in virtually everybody, with 5–15% of healthy subjects being in the abnormal range. The prevalence of rheumatoid factor seropositivity increases with age, although values are usually < 20–40 international units (or < 1/320 titre) in these patients. About 70–80% of patients with rheumatoid arthritis are seropositive (even less early in the disease). Other diseases commonly associated with rheumatoid factors are listed below.

Rheumatoid arthritis
Sjögren's syndrome
SLE
Systemic sclerosis
Subacute bacterial endocarditis
Sarcoidosis
Chronic liver disease
Polymyositis
Acute viral infections
Parasitic infections
Tuberculosis
Syphilis

Anti-nuclear antibodies (ANA)

This is not a 'lupus' test. This test should be ordered only when there are at least three other criteria for SLE. Patients should NOT be told they might have lupus just because the ANA test is positive.

ANAs are a heterogenous group which bind to nuclear antigens. When positive, this phenomenon is not specific for SLE, since it can be positive in normal subjects (5–30%, particularly in the elderly, especially when those elderly have other chronic, nonrheumatic diseases). Other conditions with positive ANA are listed below.

SLE
Systemic sclerosis
Sjögren's syndrome
Mixed connective tissue disease
Polymyositis/dermatomyositis
Idiopathic pulmonary fibrosis
Acute viral infections
Chronic active hepatitis
Diabetes mellitus

Although high titers of ANA tend to be associated with disease states, normal subjects can have high titers as well. Thus, it is very important to have a clinical suspicion for the rheumatic disease before interpreting the significance of a positive ANA.

If the ANA is positive and one does suspect the patient has a rheumatic disease, this may be further supported by detecting the specific antibody components of the ANA. Some of them are not detected in normal patients and rarely in other diseases, so are highly specific. They include antibody to double-stranded DNA (dsDNA) and anti-Sm antibodies seen in SLE, anti-Jo-1 (RNA synthetase) and anti-PM-1 (nucleolar protein) antibodies seen in polymyositis and dermatomyositis, anti-centromere antibody seen in the CREST subset of systemic sclerosis, and anti-Scl-70 (topoisomerase) antibody seen in systemic sclerosis.

Although these components are not always specific individually, specificity is increased by the otherwise negative profile for other components. For instance, a negative profile for all components of the ANA except anti-RNP (ribonucleoprotein) antibody is often seen in what is sometimes referred to as mixed connective tissue disease (MCTD). (Some believe that MCTD is not a separate entity, but that most of these patients will go on to develop scleroderma or SLE.) *Table 1.9* demonstrates the otherwise limited specificity of other individual serologic tests.

Table 1.9 Serologic tests that have multiple associations with rheumatic diseases

Antibody	Disease associations
Anti-RNP	SLE, MCTD, Sjögren's
Anti-nucleolar	Systemic sclerosis, Sjögren's
Anti-Ro/SSA	SLE, Sjögren's, neonatal SLE
Anti-La/SSB	SLE, Sjögren's, neonatal SLE

Anti-phospholipid antibodies

Indications for ordering tests for anti-phospholipid antibodies are a young patient who develops a venous or arterial thrombosis, or who develops a stroke, and women who have had repeated spontaneous abortions. Anti-phospholipid antibodies may be playing a role in some of these patients and treatment is sometimes offered on that basis. A number of diseases and complications are associated with these antibodies (see *Tables 1.10* and *1.11*).

These tests should not be ordered routinely since anti-phospholipid antibodies have been found in normal subjects, usually women, and a number of rheumatic and nonrheumatic diseases, their significance being unclear in these populations. Anti-phospholipid antibodies include the lupus anti-coagulant, anti-cardiolipin antibodies, and others. The term anti-phospholipid syndrome is used to designate a constellation of complications associated with these antibodies in the

Table 1.10 Diseases associated with anti-phospholipid antibodies

SLE
Rheumatoid arthritis
Systemic sclerosis
Polymyositis/dermatomyositis
Drugs (procainamide, hydralazine, phenytoin)
Granulomatous infections, viral infections
Hematologic malignancies
Primary anti-phospholipid syndrome

Table 1.11 Complications associated with anti-phospholipid antibodies

Venous thrombosis (any part of venous system)
Arterial thrombosis (transient ischemic attacks (TIAs), stroke, multi-infarct dementia)
Placental infarction (at any time in pregnancy)
Thrombocytopenia, hemolytic anemia
Mitral and aortic valve disease, atrial thrombi, coronary disease
(?)Guillain-Barre syndrome, transverse myelitis
(?)Global amnesia
Avascular necrosis
Pulmonary hypertension
Livedo reticularis

presence of few or no clinical manifestations of other rheumatic diseases. The anti-phospholipid antibodies may also be associated with false positive VDRL syphilis tests, and prolonged partial thromboplastin time (PTT) or prothrombin time (PT) not corrected by the addition of normal plasma.

Therapies sometimes used after patients have been identified with complications from the anti-phospholipids antibodies include control of the associated disease, as well as numerous others including ASA, corticosteroids, azathioprine, full dose heparin, warfarin (with PT international normalized ratio (INR) maintained at 3–4), immunoglobulin infusions, and plasma exchange. Some advocate the use of prophylactic corticosteroids if the patient has a history of fetal loss. There are no controlled trials to support any of these measures. Also, it is not known whether or not a patient identified as having an anti-phospholipid antibody, but not yet a clinical event, should receive prophylaxis.

Anti-neutrophil cytoplasmic antibodies (ANCAs)

One should only order tests for ANCAs after having clear evidence that some organ is being affected by a vasculitis syndrome. ANCA is reported as either p-ANCA (perinuclear staining cytoplasmic antibody) or c-ANCA (diffuse staining cytoplasmic antibody). The p-ANCA is neither a particularly sensitive nor specific test, and is of little clinical value. It is seen in Wegener's granulomatosis as well as number of other diseases (*Table 1.12*). On the other hand, c-ANCA has > 90% sensitivity for and specificity for Wegener's granulomatosus. ANCAs are rarely found in healthy subjects.

Table 1.12 Diseases associated with positive p-ANCA

Wegener's granulomatosus
Goodpasture's syndrome
Microscopic polyarteritis nodosa
Polyarteritis nodosa
Churg-Strauss vasculitis
Tuberculosis
Malaria
Leptospirosis
Amebiasis

DOs and DON'Ts of Serology

DO order serology when the clinical information from the history and physical examination meets a number of diagnostic criteria, and one wishes to confirm the diagnosis of rheumatoid arthritis or SLE.

DO explain to patients that an ANA is not strictly a 'lupus test' since many healthy subjects have a positive ANA.

DON'T order serology if a patient presents with fatigue, shoulder pain, back pain, joint pain without visible swelling, but none of the symptoms or signs listed in the diagnostic criteria of SLE, and no Raynaud's phenomenon. The patient does not have SLE, and finding a positive ANA or rheumatoid factor in this setting is of no help.

DON'T order anti-phospholipid antibody tests for every patient who has a deep venous thrombosis or miscarriage. Inevitably, some positive findings will occur and may have no significance in these patients. Order them for the patient with a clinical syndrome (multiple thromboses or miscarriages, or SLE) for which a positive finding has greater significance.

Section 2 – Diffuse pain

Top part of the algorithm

Let us begin with the patient who complains of pain and who, upon further questioning has diffuse pain (like whole arm pain). The algorithm reveals that the possibilities are:

chronic pain syndromes
polymyalgia rheumatica
malignancy.

To make the diagnosis refer to the following two topics on the first two considerations.

What about malignancy? How can one be absolutely sure that the patient does not have cancer, and at what age does one even consider this possibility? Malignancy that causes diffuse pain usually does so through bone metastases or is a hematologic malignancy, and so one expects other signs of disease. Ask about weight loss, anorexia, fever, and history of known malignancy. If any of these are present, then one must look hard for a malignancy. It is impossible for an age 'cut-off' to be made, but realize that in all aspects of medicine we rely partly on probabilities. The patient who sounds and looks as if they have fibromyalgia, who has no weight loss, no anorexia, is young, etc., has fibromyalgia. There are a few additional clues that can add some assurance (discussed below), but this is the extent to which most rheumatologists lead their diagnostic search.

Patients with chronic pain syndromes have a chronic illness; thus statistically, one expects such patients to develop cancer or coronary artery disease at the normal rate. They may present again complaining of what sounds like the same chronic aches and pains, but this time it is the bone pain of metastases or angina. There often are distinguishing features, but it is perhaps inevitable that such a diagnosis could be missed. Different physicians have different philosophies on how to deal with this dilemma.

Section 2 – Diffuse pain

Chronic pain syndromes

If a patient makes statements like those below consider a chronic pain syndrome:

I hurt all over, my fingers swell so much I can't wear my rings, and there are times when it feels like a knife is tearing through the muscles in my back.

About 13 months ago I was driving through an intersection when someone turned into me. Ever since that accident I have had incredible neck pain, every day, that goes down both my arms, and into my head as if it is going to explode. I haven't been able to work since.

I have figured out I have either lupus or Lyme disease, but I'm not sure which. (This is more likely to be said by an American patient.)

I was doing my work as I usually do as a secretary, when I lost all feeling in my arm, and by that night my entire arm was swollen to twice its size.

You know what, just sitting here while you were talking to me, I have now developed an incredible headache up the back of my skull.

Algorithmic Approach

The patient complains of pain in the shoulders and hands, and that there is occasional swelling in the hands, involving a number of joints. Now one moves down the algorithm into the arthritis zone; but this is wrong. Is her pain really localized, or is it her whole arms, neck, back of head, jaws, back, and legs? Has the swelling been observed, or was the patient's word taken for it?

The patient has diffuse pain and no swelling. So instead we move up the algorithm. She must have one of: chronic pain syndrome; polymyalgia rheumatica; or malignancy.

The diagnosis of chronic pain syndrome is confirmed by asking for more of the symptoms discussed below, and looking for tender points. The ESR is normal. The patient is rescued from the arthritis zone.

The chronic pain syndromes remain a controversial topic, particularly in the aspects of etiology and the optimal form of therapy. The comments below on these represent the authors' opinion, although such opinion is shared by many.

Chronic pain syndromes are common afflictions, and are too often misdiagnosed as arthritis, 'lupus', tendinitis, bursitis, carpal tunnel syndrome, 'pinched nerves and loose discs.' Patients receive inappropriate investigations as a response by the physician (often fueled by the patient) that 'something must be wrong for it to hurt this much.' The physician is constantly worried that he or she has missed something and hopes that the latest imaging technique or serology will reveal a tangible diagnosis and cure.

The syndrome is one chiefly characterized by the combination of unrelenting, chronic pain that may follow a trivial or minor injury (symptoms of which would normally resolve in most individuals), with no structural or pathological cause for the pain, in a patient who has abnormal behavioural and psychosocial response to pain and the 'sick role', producing an inability to cope. It is to be distinguished from a patient, for instance, who has true destructive osteoarthritis of the knee, producing chronic pain. These individuals do not develop the diffuse pain pattern of chronic pain syndromes. They learn to cope with their pain, and prefer not to adopt the 'sick role' or look for compensation. They do not organize their life around their pain.

The pain of chronic pain syndromes often moves around, and is described as 'excruciating', 'searing', 'like a knife twisting in my muscle', etc. Patients often remark on their ability to have a high pain tolerance, and for having learned to live with the pain. Paresthesias in the limbs, pain about the jaw, headaches, and irritable bowel syndrome are common complaints. Patients will often describe arthritis and joint swelling, although when viewed by a physician, no evidence of arthritis (true synovitis) can be found. They may even complain of joint stiffness, again in the absence of objective synovitis.

A common finding is abnormal sleep patterns, clinically evident by patients complaining of morning fatigue, 'unrestful sleep', and 'light' sleep. Some may describe that their bodies are fatigued and want to sleep, but that their mind does not. It is unclear, however, whether this poor 'quality' of sleep is involved in the pathogenesis or is simply a result of the chronic pain syndromes.

The original descriptions of chronic pain syndromes date back to the 1700s, when patients suffered from 'the vapours'. Following this, the diagnostic label changed to neurasthenia, then muscular rheumatism, then lumbago, and fibrositis, fibromyalgia, myofascial pain syndrome, repetitive strain injury, chronic fatigue syndrome, chronic candidiasis, and finally the all encompassing total environmental allergy syndrome. It is ironic that we have come full circle and are now diagnosing environmental 'vapours' as the cause of chronic pain syndromes again.

It is only recently that physicians are realizing that there is a psychological and behavioural response of the patient that generates and perpetuates chronic pain. We have spent more than 200 years debating controversy and searching for nonexistent pathology.

These patients commonly have a background of marital disorder, disenchanting work, financial stresses, family tragedies, and a personal history of physical, emotional, or sexual abuse. They develop abnormal pain responses and present their package of problems (manifest as a chronic pain syndrome) to the physician, hoping (subconsciously) that a solution lies within the physician's medical acumen. 'There must be some cause for all this pain, particularly being so severe,' they reason. There is, it just isn't structural or pathological – it is behavioral and psychological. There is no medication that corrects these problems, but the patient must have insight into how these factors affect their outcome – inability to obtain such insight leads to a poor prognosis.

These patients get to a point in their life when they 'can't cope', until finally a chronic pain develops. This chronic pain syndrome offers a tangible reason for being helpless rather than 'inability to cope' and to maintain control of their problems. The 'sick role' offers an escape, even if the patient does not realize it, and pursuit of disease by the medical profession reinforces this escape.

Physicians reinforce the pain pattern by doing unnecessary investigations. Patients proceed on the logical assumption that if the physician is doing investigations, he or she must think there is some disease present, otherwise they would not do the investigation. When a patient is referred to another physician for a diagnosis, this further reinforces the concept that a specific disease must be present. Following a series of inconclusive investigations providing irrelevant data, a series of referrals to physiotherapists, chiropractors, rheumatologists, neurologists, surgeons, etc., a long period (often years) of frustration for both the patient and the primary care physician is maintained. Incredible costs due to laboratory investigations, referrals, ineffective medications, and loss of time off work, compensation benefits, and disability pensions ensue.

Some of the defined forms of chronic pain syndromes include fibromyalgia, regional myofascial pain syndrome, repetitive strain injury, and chronic fatigue syndrome. They are discussed below. There is tremendous clinical overlap, however, between the different forms of chronic pain syndromes, and one may not be able to always label a patient with one term. One should not become pre-occupied with classification schemes in chronic pain syndromes, since it is often disappointing to find how much disagreement there is between clinicians who see these patients, and how conflicting the literature can be on this subject.

Diagnosis

One should consider a chronic pain syndrome as number one on the differential diagnosis when the statements described above are made. The history is so useful in these illnesses, that it should be a relatively easy task to make the diagnosis.

Everyone is worried about missing something serious. There really are no diseases which can produce all the symptoms and signs these patients have. Rheumatologists are very good at diagnosing these conditions, not because they are brilliant, but rather out of simplicity. They cannot think of another illness that possibly explains this patient's symptoms.

First, look at the whole package the patient presents. Do not focus immediately on each symptom. Rather than thinking, 'Oh, the patient has hand numbness; now what are the questions that I need to ask about carpal tunnel syndrome', take a few minutes to ask some leading questions. In the patient who really has only carpal tunnel syndrome, there is no loss in asking these questions and finding out that the responses are negative. One can then focus on the presenting complaint.

Ask a few questions like, 'I understand that you have numbness, but tell me, do you have any pains anywhere?' 'Anywhere else? 'And what about headaches?' 'And what about pain in your neck region?' 'And what about pain over your jaw?' 'And what about your sleep, what's that like?' 'Are you tired?' After the answers to these questions are positive, then ask yourself if you believe carpal tunnel syndrome explains these symptoms – of course it does not.

Ask about weight loss. It is such a rare event that it should be an important clue to something serious. The patient may have clinical depression, or if they are elderly may have a malignancy.

Finally, for complete reassurance, review the algorithm described in Section 1 'Approach to rheumatic diseases' (*Figure 1.1*, page 2). Look for symptoms and signs one would seek in the diagnosis of rheumatoid arthritis, SLE, seronegative spondyloarthropathy, etc. Consider diseases like polymyalgia rheumatica and giant cell arteritis in the elderly patient. If none of these features are present or there are too few criteria to even entertain diagnoses like rheumatoid arthritis, SLE, etc., no further investigations are required (i.e. no serology, no X-rays). Proceed with explaining chronic pain syndrome to the patient.

One should be careful not to routinely order serology tests such as for rheumatoid factor or ANA when a patient presents with symptoms typical of chronic pain. Too often, patients with fibromyalgia are told they may have SLE because they were found to have a positive ANA. One SHOULD NOT order serologic tests for a patient who complains of joint aches or pains, but does not have other criteria to suggest the diagnosis of rheumatoid arthritis or SLE.

One should not confuse paresthesias these patients sometimes have with carpal tunnel syndrome. If the patient lacks the typical nocturnal episodes of awakening with pain or numbness that is relieved by violent shaking out of the hands, then they have virtually no chance of having carpal tunnel syndrome. Although carpal tunnel symptoms may become nearly constant, they should have started with these nocturnal symptoms. As well, carpal tunnel syndrome does not cause palpable tenderness and tender points. Thus, the vast majority of patients with chronic pain syndromes and paresthesias **DO NOT** require nerve conduction studies.

Treatment

It is important to be honest with the patient right from the beginning, and tell them not to focus on investigations or referrals, or dependency on a physiotherapist. The patients must be told that if they want their condition to improve they will have to take on the responsibility of therapy; that is, continued use and exercise of the affected region. Too often the burden of 'cure' is placed in the wrong hands; the physician's.

1. Tell the patient that they have a chronic pain syndrome, and that their history and findings confirm this rather than some other diagnosis. There are many terms given to such syndromes, including muscular rheumatism, fibrositis, fibromyalgia, chronic fatigue syndrome, etc.

2. Reassure the patient they do not have a form of arthritis, rheumatoid arthritis, SLE, or other serious joint-damaging diseases. No matter how painful their condition is, it will never cause joint, nerve, or muscle damage, even when activity seems painful.

3. The chronic pain syndromes are of unknown cause, even though they have been around for a few hundred years at least. Studies have shown no evidence of tissue damage, in any case, in any of these conditions.

4. Tell them their pain is very real, and chronic pain syndromes can exist even when there is not something like tendinitis, or muscle or joint disease.

5. We do not know why someone gets such chronic pain, but we do know that we can identify risk factors common to patients with chronic pain syndromes. Ask about personal relationships, work history, family and any financial difficulties, or recent tragic events for the patient. Don't just ask the patient if they have any stresses (most will say no), but instead ask about the various aspects of their life and you will encounter the patient's various problems. Tell them that psychosocial factors are not necessarily the cause of the pain, but clearly may have 'set them up' for developing a chronic pain syndrome, by mechanisms we do not yet understand. Some physicians use the analogy of phantom limb pain to explain how someone can have perception of pain when there is no structural reason. (Phantom limb pain is pain in a limb that is no longer there.)

6. Explain to the patient that narcotic analgesics are not useful, and that only in a few are NSAIDs helpful. Consider offering medications to improve sleep (amitriptyline 25–75 mg qhs), imipramine, nortriptyline, trazodone, doxepin (all 10–50 mg qhs), and fluoxetine (20 mg qd), but remind the patient that there is no medication that is going to cure this problem, only help with therapy. DO NOT prescribe narcotics or benzodiazepines no matter how much pain the patient is experiencing.

7. Do not feel (or let the patient make you feel) that you have failed if you cannot offer a cure to the patient. Do not be pressed into starting medication or ordering tests because the patient insists you try to find a cause. It is much better for the patient, and more cost-effective, to tell them that a second opinion to confirm the chronic pain syndrome (not to find a diagnosis, because you have a diagnosis) is more worthwhile than unnecessary investigations.

   If the patient insists on a referral, send them to a physician who is competent in diagnosing chronic pain syndromes. (Rheumatologists are often asked to see such patients, and can diagnose their condition without further investigations, at the same time reassuring the patient.) The physician will confirm the diagnosis of a chronic pain syndrome, and help make it clear to the patient that no further investigations are needed. This is preferable to spending a few months treating with NSAIDs, then analgesics, then physiotherapy, then more investigations, etc. Diagnose chronic pain syndromes early, and if the patient does not accept that diagnosis, refer to another physician who will give the patient that second opinion they want, and confirm your diagnosis.

8. Do not let the patient focus and become obsessed with the fact that their neck X-ray shows degenerative changes, etc. X-ray changes are not well correlated with symptoms, and such findings never explain a chronic pain syndrome. Be straightforward and honest with the patient that the X-ray findings may actually be irrelevant.

9. Some patients will change physicians when they are not satisfied that enough investigations are being done. They will inevitably encounter one who tells them they have arthritis, and need many more investigations. The patient will be happy with this and have the 'sick role' reinforced. You cannot prevent the incompetence of that physician, but you can at least know you are not part of the problem.

10. Tell the patient quite honestly that they (not others) may be able to cure their pain, but the real goal of therapy is to improve function and coping. The patient must understand that they have to work and remain active when in pain, or they will develop further problems. One does not wait until the pain is completely gone before deciding on readiness for work. The pain may never go away! The patient cannot be allowed to stop working indefinitely. If there is any period of 'sick-leave' it should only be

for a few weeks, and the patient should return to work even if they continue to have pain.

11. Chronic pain syndromes are not truly physically disabling. This is evidenced by the fact that farmers or self-employed individuals with no other financial resources who have developed chronic pain syndromes (even with severe symptoms) rarely alter their work pattern (because they would otherwise lose the farm). Yet many workers in various jobs where compensation is available complain that they cannot possibly work. If a disease is physically disabling, it should be indiscriminate of work circumstances.

If a patient with multiple sclerosis and leg weakness, for example, is asked to do heavy labor in a warehouse, as a heavy duty mechanic, or as a farmer, they will have difficulty with any of these jobs. The farmer may try a lot harder to keep working, but will eventually have to alter his or her work pattern. Multiple sclerosis is a disabling disease. An individual with a chronic pain syndrome, may complain that he or she cannot work as a heavy duty mechanic, but a self-employed farmer will continue to work despite the chronic pain syndrome. This incongruity between the way a chronic pain syndrome can be disabling for some types of physical labor and not others is the reason why chronic pain syndromes are not true physical disabilities. Farmers prove every day that patients with chronic pain syndromes (no matter how severe the symptoms) can continue to perform difficult physical labor.

12. Regular exercise and return to work is the best form of therapy. The response of the patient to the advice of engaging in exercise even if on a slow gradual build-up of capacity, is often that such an endeavor is impossible because they are too tired and in too much pain to do so. If a patient will have pain and fatigue all the time anyway, they may as well choose to experience it during exercise once a day as well. At least then they have the benefit of exercise, and no loss because they were going to have pain at rest in any case.

13. Have the patient return for another visit to review and reinforce this education.

The duration of chronic pain syndromes is quite variable. While some say such illnesses often resolve in a few years, and tell patients this, many rheumatologists have diagnosed patients with chronic pain syndromes and encountered them again 10 years later with the same or similar complaints. The patient who stops working because of their symptoms, recurrent depression, poor social relationships, anxiety disorder, long history (many years) of chronic pain syndrome, chronic headaches or irritable bowel syndrome, obesity, and no insight into the fact that these factors may be related to their illness tend to do poorly. There is no medication that can correct all of these factors.

Fibromyalgia

Fibromyalgia is also sometimes referred to as fibrositis (a misnomer, given the lack of evidence for inflammation) and pain magnification syndrome. The most important physical findings include classic tender points. The nine symmetric pairs of sites (total = 18) are shown in *Figure 2.1*. The specificity of these tender points for fibromyalgia is increased by finding at least 11 points. It is said that the pressure applied should be about 4 kg, but most physicians recognize what degree of pressure does not cause pain in normal subjects.

The patient should have their complaints of pain present for at least 3 months, and should have pain in both the right and left, and the upper and lower regions of the body. Their complaint of pain in these regions is important, since one may encounter patients who have the classic tender points, but no complaints of pain there normally. The best example of this is in rheumatoid arthritis, where perhaps 50% of patients have the tender points of fibromyalgia, but have no complaints of pain there otherwise. Most rheumatoid arthritis patients are not treated for fibromyalgia in the conventional sense, and yet can remain free of fibromyalgia symptoms. It may be possible, however, that the expression of

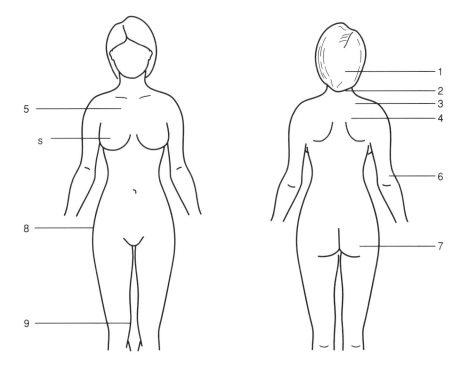

Fig. 2.1 The nine symmetric tender points of fibromyalgia. (1) Suboccipital muscle insertion; (2) Low cervical; (3) Trapezius; (4) Supraspinatus origins; (5) Second costochondral junctions; (6) Lateral humeral condyles – 2 cm distal; (7) Gluteal; (8) Greater femoral trochanters; (9) Medial fat pads of the knee. S, Silicon breast implant.

these tender points may be in the form of fatigue or promoting disuse for reasons which the patient may be unaware. The significance of finding such tender points in rheumatoid arthritis is unclear.

It is possible, however, for patients with rheumatoid arthritis, polymyositis, and polymyalgia rheumatica, for example, also to complain of diffuse pain, with the finding of classic tender points. Assuming other measures of the primary disease are clearly responding to therapy (i.e. synovitis in rheumatoid arthritis, muscle strength and creatinine kinase (CK) in polymyositis, and stiffness and ESR in polymyalgia rheumatica), it is reasonable to also diagnose fibromyalgia in this setting.

Examination should otherwise reveal normal muscle strength, or, occasionally, give-way weakness. The CK level and ESR should be normal. Some argue that the serum thyroid stimulating hormone level should be checked because hypothyroidism can present in this fashion. It is also recommended that if an elderly patient presents with what seems to be fibromyalgia, one should consider malignancy (and in particular hypercalcemia due to the malignancy) as a cause since fibromyalgia is less common in this age group.

Repetitive strain syndrome

This diagnosis has appeared and is now disappearing after the Australian government learned it was an illness whose incidence depended on how easily financial workers' compensation could be obtained. Individuals whose occupation included repetitive activity were reported to have developed chronic pain syndromes, usually in the arms. Patients complained of swelling where none was actually found. Poor grip strength due to pain and paresthesias often developed. On examination, there is no clear-cut swelling of painful regions, and a normal neurologic examination (or apparent sensory loss does not entirely conform to anatomic nerve distribution). The therapy is much like that for any chronic pain syndrome, but the prognosis is poor if the patient stops using the limb, the pain often lasting for months to years. In particular, there often are complicating issues of compensation claims.

Regional myofascial pain syndrome

This illness often produces pain and tenderness in a specific region (e.g. arm, right trapezius, whole hand) with no prior history of trauma or specific repetitive use. It is clear how this illness may relate to fibromyalgia, and certainly patients can have some of the classic tender points. There may be complaints of fatigue and sleep disturbance. They may also complain of subjective soft tissue swelling. If they at some point have had physician-documented swelling of the affected limb, then think immediately of reflex sympathetic dystrophy (see page 175).

Chronic fatigue syndrome

This syndrome may also be related to fibromyalgia, since soft tissue pain and tenderness is seen, but the most prominent symptom is debilitating fatigue > 6 months. The patient may also have low-grade fever, sore throat, painful lymph nodes (< 2 cm), headaches, migratory arthralgias without arthritis, and sleep disturbance. One should do a complete history and physical examination in these individuals to look for causes of fatigue, considering common ones like depression, lifestyle stresses, hypothyroidism, anemia of any cause, malignancy, COPD, and congestive heart failure.

Temporomandibular joint dysfunction syndrome

Patients with complaints of jaw pain or headache are not usually seen in rheumatology clinics, but the illness sometimes termed temporomandibular joint dysfunction (TMJ) syndrome (also called oromandibular dysfunction) has some features that overlap with other chronic pain syndromes. This must be distinguished from temporomandibular arthritis seen uncommonly in rheumatoid arthritis, where it occurs in the setting of obvious evidence of rheumatoid arthritis elsewhere. Patients with TMJ dysfunction complain of chronic pain in the region of the jaw, ear, or neck. They describe frequent noises related to jaw motion, 'pressure in the ear', tinnitus, jaw pain with chewing, talking and yawning. They are often told they grind their teeth while sleeping. There is often an association with headaches, including migraines, sleep disorder, and fatigue.

Examination may reveal lateral jaw deviation during opening, pain over the joint, and pain over the tonsillar pillars. It is not uncommon for patients with fibromyalgia, and regional chronic pain syndromes of the upper limb to complain of similar symptoms and have similar jaw findings. Radiographs of the jaw may be abnormal, but there has been little evidence that such abnormalities are correlated with prognosis, symptoms, or response to therapy. As in other chronic pain syndromes, one would expect the ESR and CBC to be normal.

Some patients will respond to nocturnal bite plates, although there are obviously no controlled (and certainly not blinded) trials to support that this is not a placebo effect. Some will clearly fail to respond to such therapy. Others have a temporary response only. The more symptoms the patient has beyond jaw pain, the less likely it is that oral bite plates alone will help solve their problem.

Total environmental allergy syndrome of multiple chemical sensitivity

In the 18th Century this was known as the vapours – enough said.

Chronic back or neck pain (whiplash) after an accident

Another specific group of chronic pain syndromes has evolved in our system of workers' compensation and accident litigation. These patients are not usually malingering, or just trying to get some income. In fact, many times successful attainment of their financial compensation does not alleviate their chronic pain.

It is interesting that it is rare for individuals in single-vehicle accidents, or involved in accidents where they are the liable party, to get chronic pain syndromes. Such patients do get neck pain, for instance, for several days after an accident, but then the pain resolves completely. Patients who are 'innocent' in accidents somehow develop an abnormal pain behavior that cannot be explained by any structural damage.

The back or neck pain tends to be very diffuse, often constant (even at rest), described as 'severe', 'tearing of muscles', 'stabbing', or 'burning'. Neurologic examination results will be normal, although the patient may complain of paresthesias. There is no known reason why patients should be so debilitated by a motor vehicle accident that produces no structural damage, while many individuals suffer more severe injuries with actual spinal fractures, or spondylolisthesis and recover from their symptoms within weeks.

Often the patients focus on abnormalities of their spine X-rays, and point out that because their spine does not appear normal they cannot work. Remind the patient that degenerative changes are universal and appear in increasing amounts as people age, regardless of whether or not pain is present. Also, bulging discs on CT scan or MRI are irrelevant, since unless neurologic examination confirms nerve impingement, they are not a reason to stop working. Again, many of these changes are present in the general population (including 30% of young individuals) without causing symptoms, and are often present for years before any accident occurs. These patients are best treated with the reassurance that they have only a minor muscle injury, avoiding the use of collars or braces, and neck stretches (see Appendix 1), and using the same suggestions as for fibromyalgia.

Reflex sympathetic dysfunction

Some clinicians use the term 'reflex sympathetic dysfunction' or 'dystrophy' to mean any of the chronic pain syndromes. When reflex sympathetic dystrophy is referred to in this text (see page 175) it means only that entity described in rheumatology texts as characterized by an episode of true swelling with bone scan and X-ray changes typical of this disease. Do not confuse these two. One is treated with NSAID's, prednisone (prednisolone), or calcitonin (reflex sympathetic dystrophy, the one with true swelling) while the chronic pain syndromes are not.

DOs and DON'Ts of chronic pain syndromes

DO consider this diagnosis when a patient complains of diffuse aches and pains (whole body or whole limb), rather than incorrectly telling the patient they have arthritis.

DO ask patients to return when they have joint swelling so that it can be confirmed.

DO ask about and look for criteria used to diagnose SLE, rheumatoid arthritis, myositis, and tendinitis.

DO ask about weight loss and documented fever as clues to a systemic disease.

DO feel confident in making these diagnoses, and explain to the patient that they do not have SLE, arthritis, or serious tissue-damaging disease.

DO tell the patient that it is their effort that will chiefly determine prognosis, although medications sometimes help.

DO tell the patient that they will not cause tissue-damage by physical activity.

DO consider reflex sympathetic dystrophy rather than regional myofascial pain if there was a **physician-documented** episode of prolonged, diffuse swelling.

DO send the patient to work. Chronic pain syndromes are not a cause for disability, and work is frequently therapeutic for patients with chronic pain.

DON'T prescribe cervical collars, splints, or braces for chronic pain syndromes.

DON'T use lack of pain as an indicator of readiness for work (they will never be ready if this is used). Instead, be firm to allow at most a few weeks off work, and insist that the patient is not eligible for disability because patients with chronic pain syndromes must return to work for their own good, despite pain.

DON'T order serology unless you have clinical evidence of a specific disease.

DON'T order nerve conduction studies on patients with chronic pain syndromes and paresthesias. Learn to separate them from carpal tunnel syndrome, by lacking the classic nocturnal symptoms.

DON'T blindly order CT or MRI scans on patients with chronic pain syndromes, because in a small percentage you will find abnormalities that are actually irrelevant, but the patient may become obsessed with that finding as the root of their problems.

DON'T let a patient fixate on the fact that they have some abnormality on spine X-ray, since it is irrelevant to the cause of their pain.

DON'T routinely order radiologic studies on patients complaining of temporomandibular joint (TMJ) pain. There is poor correlation between symptoms and X-ray findings. A number of individuals in the general population will have abnormal results without symptoms.

DON'T treat chronic pain syndromes with narcotics or benzodiazepines.

Section 2 – Diffuse pain

Polymyalgia rheumatica

Polymyalgia rheumatica, like giant cell (or temporal) arteritis, is rare before the age of 50. The onset of symptoms is usually abrupt, with pain and stiffness in lower neck, shoulder girdle, hips, and thighs. Morning stiffness is very prominent. There are often systemic symptoms such as anorexia, malaise, fever, and weight loss. Occasionally there may be synovitis of the large joints. Twenty percent may have symptoms or signs of giant cell arteritis (see the section on vasculitis, page 168).

Algorithmic Approach

The patient complains of shoulder and back pain, with pain in the legs. You ask them to point exactly to where the pain is and it appears to be diffuse over these areas. According to the algorithm, the patient must have one of: chronic pain syndrome; polymyalgia rheumatica; or malignancy.

The chronic pain syndrome is easily excluded by the questions in the previous topic. Polymyalgia rheumatica is confirmed by an elevated ESR, morning stiffness, and asking about giant cell (temporal) arteritis symptoms. Malignancy is considered in the elderly, who usually have risk factors (e.g. smokers, known history of carcinoma), weight loss, and anorexia.

The diagnosis is based on the clinical presentation, an elevated ESR, and normal creatine kinase (CK) level. The patient may demonstrate joint restriction of movement on active testing, but not with passive testing. Unlike myositis, true muscle weakness will not be evident.

The disease must be distinguished from 'polymyalgic' onset of rheumatoid arthritis, in which the synovitis is usually more prominent, the arthritis eventually erosive, and the response to low-dose corticosteroids used for polymyalgia rheumatica usually insufficient for therapy of the arthritis. SLE may have such an onset, but is a much less common disease in the elderly, with Raynaud's phenomenon, oral ulcers, malar rash, etc. not being seen in polymyalgia rheumatica. It is very unusual for polymyalgia to produce only upper limb symptoms, since low back and thigh symptoms should also be present. If the patient's complaints are only around the shoulders, consider adhesive capsulitis (frozen shoulder), or supraspinatus tendinitis.

Polymyositis has true muscle weakness, and elevated CK level. The CK level is normal in polymyalgia rheumatica.

The treatment is prednisone (prednisolone) 15 mg qd, usually maintained for 4–6 weeks, tapering gradually to lower doses and eventually alternate-day or low-dose daily therapy. The pain of polymyalgia responds extremely well to corticosteroids. Failure to do so within a few days or a week actually suggests another diagnosis. The patient should expect to be on therapy for at least 1 year, often 2 years or more. Relapse is not uncommon, and should be treated again with 1 year of corticosteroid. A third relapse is rare. It is also worthwhile to have a rheumatologist involved to be certain of the diagnosis, since the patient is being committed to long-term corticosteroid therapy.

DOs and DON'Ts of Polymyalgia Rheumatica

DO ask about headache, acute visual loss, diplopia, and jaw pain. This suggests giant cell arteritis and warrants biopsy.

DO check to make sure no true muscle weakness exists. Confirm that the CK level is normal before concluding the patient has polymyalgia rheumatica.

DON'T use ESR alone to guide therapy. As long as the patient with polymyalgia rheumatica alone is asymptomatic, continue tapering the corticosteroid dose.

DON'T increase corticosteroid dose for nonspecific symptoms like malaise, fatigue, nausea, or generalized aches. If unsure of whether or not to increase the dose, or if a patient seems to complain of these symptoms every time the dose is lowered, consult a rheumatologist.

Section 3 – Localized pain

Middle part of the algorithm

Now we can proceed as if the patient has complained of localized pain, and there is no swelling. This brings us to the distinct possibilities of: tendinitis/bursitis; osteoarthritis; or systemic lupus erythematosus (SLE).

The most common cause of localized rheumatic pains is tendinitis/bursitis, but how do you decide which of the three possibilities is the correct diagnosis? Gathering all the detail of the patient's pain, when it occurs, and exactly what contortion reproduces their pain is not very efficient or effective in a diagnostic sense. In fact, for most regional pain complaints, there are very few questions to ask.

Instead, once this point in the algorithm has been reached, one knows that one is limiting the diagnosis considerably. For SLE (which seldom presents in this fashion in any case), ask the questions in the diagnostic criteria and that possibility will be eliminated altogether. To decide whether or not the patient has tendinitis/bursitis or osteoarthritis causing the regional pain, simply proceed with the approaches described below; a specific examination technique designed to distinguish these two possibilities.

Section 3 – Localized pain

Painful shoulder

Shoulder pain can arise from a number of sites, including the rotator cuff tendons, biceps tendon, the subacromial (subdeltoid) bursa, the glenohumeral joint, acromioclavicular joint, and the sternoclavicular joint. These sources of shoulder pain tend to produce pain either very near the shoulder joint, in the deltoid region, or over the anterior and lateral aspect of the biceps region, where it is sometimes referred. There are specific maneuvres in the examination that can isolate each of these structures and determine if it is the cause of the pain, and palpable tenderness is usually located at either only one site or in a small area. This helps to distinguish shoulder pain from these sources from chronic pain syndromes involving the shoulder region, in which case there is diffuse shoulder pain, with radiation to arm and neck, no objective loss in passive range of motion, and multiple tender points.

Algorithmic Approach

When a patient complains of shoulder pain, the first step is to determine localization since, on questioning, patients with chronic pain syndromes will be found to have pain in their neck, shoulder, arm, forearm, and hand.

Now you are traveling down the algorithm because the patient has localized their pain. Swelling in the shoulder joint is rare, except in cases of septic arthritis or pseudogout, whereby a patient will have so much shoulder pain that they and you cannot move their shoulder. The patient needs a joint aspiration if you suspect septic arthritis or pseudogout. In the absence of swelling the choices on the algorithm include: tendinitis/bursitis; osteoarthritis; and SLE.

You do not have to bother with SLE in this case, but even if you did, by proceeding through the diagnostic criteria, you would have ruled this out. So this leaves tendinitis/bursitis or osteoarthritis. Proceed now with the shoulder examination and the diagnosis will be evident.

It is very common for shoulder pain to be much worse during sleep when the source is one of the specific structures mentioned, whereas in chronic pain syndromes, this nocturnal pain is not much worse than pain during the day.

Reflex sympathetic dystrophy may also affect the shoulder, usually at the same time, producing characteristic hand swelling. Late cases of reflex sympathetic dystrophy may sometimes be difficult to separate from chronic pain syndromes, but in the former there is often objective muscle wasting, and X-rays and bone scan are abnormal (due to the development of regional osteoporosis).

The markers of a more serious disorder in the shoulder are obvious swelling (which is seen as an anterior bulging) that suggests arthritis (including infection), fever and chills, axillary pain, inability to maintain arm elevation (see later under supraspinatus tests for rotator cuff tear or atrophy, page 44), and systemic symptoms such as weight loss, anorexia, and night sweats.

One must always be aware of the fact that pain may be referred to the shoulder from other sites in the chest, neck, or abdomen, in which case shoulder examination will be normal.

Examination of the shoulder

Examination of the shoulder is key to the diagnosis. A concise and practical examination method is described here. This has to be modified for some very specific orthopedic or neurologic diseases, but will suffice for the diagnosis of most shoulder disorders.

Normal ranges of motion are:

Abduction	90°
Internal rotation	90°
External rotation	90°
Flexion	180°
Extension	60°

The examination proceeds through the stages listed below.

1. Start with the patient seated. Look at both shoulders anteriorly for their normal contours. Observe if there is any difference in appearance between the two shoulders that may indicate swelling, bony dislocation, or muscle atrophy. Then look over the scapula and view the supraspinatus muscle occupying the upper part of the scapula, and the infraspinatus occupying the lower part of the scapula (*Figure 3.1*). Normally the muscle bulk of these muscles provides a rounded surface to the scapular region. Flattening or concavity of these muscles suggests either rotator muscle atrophy or rotator cuff tear. Elderly patients may often have flattening of the contour of this muscle, which may not be significant in this age group.

2. Ask the patient to point with one finger to the source of pain. A wide sweep of the hand, particularly tracing down the arm and up to the neck is almost never seen in tendinitis, but is common in chronic pain syndromes.

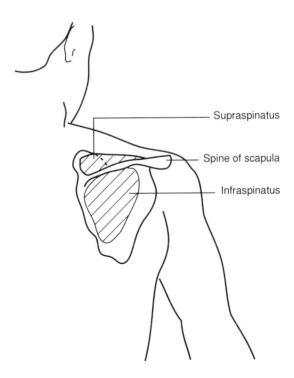

Fig. 3.1 The supraspinatus and infraspinatus muscles.

The pain of rotator cuff (supraspinatus, infraspinatus, subscapularis) tendinitis or biceps tendinitis is usually right over the shoulder or over the upper biceps and triceps muscles.

3. Then examine the abduction arcs to determine whether or not the pain is originating from rotator cuff tendinitis or from the shoulder joints (glenohumeral, sternoclavicular, and acromioclavicular). Have the patient place their arms at their sides while standing, and ask them to slowly abduct them eventually bringing their arms above their heads with palms facing each other. Ask the patient to indicate whether there is pain at any point during this arc of abduction, when it starts and when it stops. In supraspinatus (or rotator cuff) tendinitis the pain will begin at around 60° from the body and continue until 120° where it then becomes less as the patient brings their hands together with palms facing each other. This is impingement syndrome or 'rotator cuff syndrome' associated with tendinitis (see below).

If, however, the patient begins to feel pain at 90–120° and continues to feel pain with further abduction to putting their palms together, there is one of acromioclavicular, sternoclavicular, or glenohumeral arthritis present (*Figure 3.2*). One can confirm impingement syndrome by 'impingement

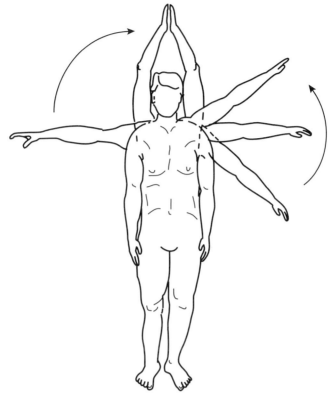

Fig. 3.2 The painful arcs of abduction.

tests' (*Figures 3.3* and *3.4*), and arthritis by palpating that joint specifically (see below).

4. If the patient cannot complete the abduction motion due to weakness, passively place the arm in 90° abduction. Now forward flex the arm 30°, and rotate it internally so that the thumb is pointing down (*Figure 3.5*). This isolates the supraspinatus tendon. Now ask the patient to slowly lower the arm to their side. If the arm drops suddenly, they have a rotator cuff tear or significant muscle atrophy producing this weakness. An arthrogram or MRI will differentiate between these two easily.

5. Having completed the abduction arcs, check internal rotation (which reveals glenohumeral disorders including adhesive capsulitis) and external rotation (tendinitis, and often adhesive capsulitis). Have the patient place their arms behind their back and attempt to place their hand as high up towards their scapula as they can (*Figure 3.6*). This tests internal rotation, and normally the thumbs should reach the inferior aspects of the scapulae. Pain with or restriction of this motion is seen in glenohumeral arthritis and adhesive

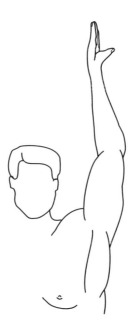

Fig. 3.3 An impingement test (passively forward flex 180°, internally rotate shoulder).

capsulitis (frozen shoulder). Patients with more severe cases of supraspinatus tendinitis can have pain with internal rotation because slight abduction
is required to place the hand behind the back. One should have already
determined from the abduction arc and impingement tests whether or not
supraspinatus tendinitis exists, however, and should bear this in mind when
the patient is asked to internally rotate and put their hand behind their back.

To test external rotation have the patient place their elbows at their sides,
with elbows flexed at 90°. Ask them to move their forearms outward (see
Figure 3.7) to test for infraspinatus tendinitis, or adhesive capsulitis (frozen
shoulder). Infraspinatus tendinitis produces pain on external rotation, but
normal range. Adhesive capsulitis produces pain and limited range of external rotation.

6. You have now determined which abduction arc was painful (both may have
    been), and whether or not internal rotation was abnormal (glenohumeral
    arthritis or adhesive capsulitis), or external rotation was abnormal (tendinitis
    or adhesive capsulitis).

To test for biceps tendinitis, have the patient flex at the shoulder to bring
their arm (elbow extended) forward and upward to nearly 180°. Then have
the patient make the same movement with resistance applied to the arm
just above the elbow. Pain with resistance may represent biceps tendinitis,
but sometimes other sources will cause pain with this maneuver, thus some

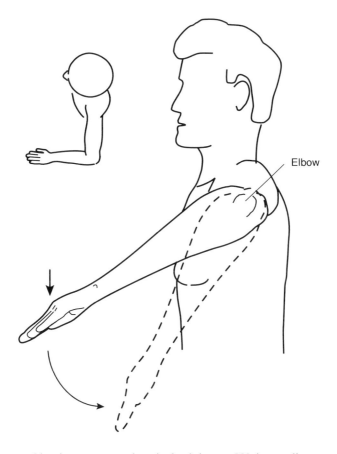

Fig. 3.4 A second impingement test (passively abduct to 90°, internally rotate shoulder).

patients are over-diagnosed with biceps tendinitis. Palpation over the biceps tendon should be done as well (see step 8) to confirm this diagnosis.

7. If the patient does not have full active movement with any of these maneuvers, passively test the range. If the range becomes normal as you test it, then the patient has tendinitis. If the passive range of motion is also abnormal, then there is a joint disorder.

8. Finally, palpate the shoulder region (*Figure 3.8*). Start with the sternoclavicular joint which cannot only cause shoulder pain, but pain with movement as the clavicle must rotate at this joint when the shoulder moves. Then palpate the length of the clavicle to note any crepitus which may indicate a fracture. As you proceed laterally along the clavicle, you will encounter a bony prominence, this being the acromioclavicular joint, which should be palpated. Then place the arm in internal rotation (put the patient's hand behind their back) and right below the acromioclavicular joint on the anterior convexity of the humeral head is the greater tuberosity (*Figure 3.9*).

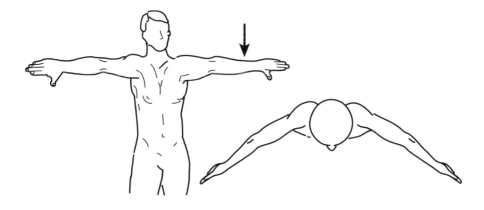

Fig. 3.5 The supraspinatus (drop-arm) test for rotator cuff tear or atrophy.

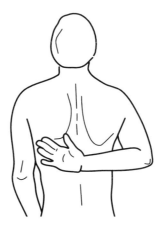

Fig. 3.6 Test for internal rotation (or glenerohumeral arthritis or adhesive capsulitis).

This is tender when the patient has supraspinatus tendinitis (this is where the muscle inserts). About 1 cm medial to the greater tuberosity is the biceps groove, and this is tender in biceps tendinitis.

Key examination points

- Painful arcs of abduction indicate tendinitis (60°–120°) or arthritis (90°–180°).
- Restricted internal rotation suggests a glenohumeral joint disorder (arthritis or adhesive capsulitis).

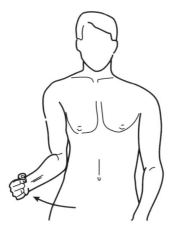

Fig. 3.7   Test of external rotation (infraspinatus tendinitis or adhesive capsulitis).

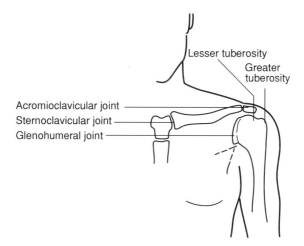

Fig. 3.8   Three joints of the shoulder.

- External rotation is restricted early in adhesive capsulitis (frozen shoulder).
- If there is restricted active movement, check passive movement. Passive range of movement improves in tendinitis, but not in arthritis or adhesive capsulitis.

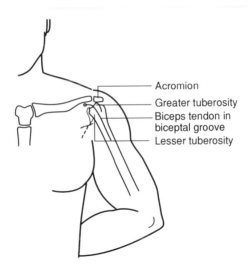

Acromion
Greater tuberosity
Biceps tendon in
biceptal groove
Lesser tuberosity

Fig. 3.9 Palpation of the greater tuberosity for supraspinatus tendinitis.

The diagnosis and management of some specific shoulder disorders are discussed below, emphasizing again historical or physical features that aid in diagnosis. Physiotherapy exercises for shoulder disorders are described in Appendix 1.

Impingement syndrome (supraspinatus or rotator cuff tendinitis)

This is a common cause of shoulder pain in inflammatory arthropathies, sports injuries, and occupational injuries. It is sometimes referred to as a rotator cuff syndrome. It occurs when the supraspinatus tendon of the rotator cuff and the subacromial (subdeltoid) bursa are 'caught' between the humeral head and the coracoacromial ligament, and produces supraspinatus tendinitis, and subacromial (subdeltoid) bursitis. This may result from overuse injuries of the supraspinatus tendon (e.g. in athletes or workers). In patients with a primary condition such as rheumatoid arthritis or osteoarthritis of the glenohumeral joint, chronic inflammation and disuse leads to rotator cuff atrophy. Presumably, the now less-opposed activity of the deltoid muscle pulls the humeral head upward into a position in which impingement is more likely to occur.

By either cause, the patient will complain of pain during the arc of abduction from 60° to 120° (or more often pain with activities that require arm abduction, (e.g. combing the hair, reaching above the shoulder level, etc.)). They may also have pain at rest and especially at night from secondary supraspinatus tendinitis and subacromial bursitis that develops or worsens with chronic impingement. The patient may complain of pain over the shoulder and the upper arm muscles. Repeated injury to the tendon leads to disuse, further attrition, and perhaps rotator cuff atrophy or tear.

Examination will reveal localization of pain anteriorly or laterally, and perhaps supraspinatus muscle atrophy as visualized over the scapula. The patient will develop pain with active abduction, with the pain improving as the arm is abducted beyond 120°. Shoulder flexion and extension are usually not affected (but may be if there is a primary arthropathy). The pain can be reproduced with impingement tests.

Radiographs may show a subacromial spur, small amounts of tendon calcification, sclerosis of the greater tuberosity at the supraspinatus tendon insertion, and rotator cuff atrophy (the vertical height between the humeral head and the overlying acromium in anteroposterior view should be at least 10 mm normally; less indicating atrophy of the rotator cuff).

Therapy is directed at avoiding the specific maneuvers that cause impingement, maintaining shoulder range of motion, NSAIDs, physiotherapy, and occasionally corticosteroid injection into the bursa or region of the rotator cuff. The corticosteroid injection should be avoided in injury-related impingement since presumably most cases can be resolved with conservative therapy, and there is a small risk of further atrophy or rupture with repeated injections. In patients with rheumatoid arthritis, who have a chronic inflammatory disorder, the above should be tried, but corticosteroid injections are more often used, as they more often have refractory cases.

Surgery is used in moderate to complete rotator cuff tears, or refractory cases. This is particularly true in athletes. In patients with rheumatoid arthritis, however, or those with considerable rotator cuff atrophy, there is often no surgical option.

Calcific supraspinatus tendinitis

Supraspinatus tendinitis may sometimes be accompanied by significant hydroxyapatite deposits in the tendon, and bursa. It tends to present as a very acute attack of shoulder pain mimicking pseudogout. Radiographs show significant calcification in the tendon or bursa (minor 'specks' of calcification are sometimes seen in chronic impingement syndrome described above), and this is the only real distinguishing feature from ordinary rotator cuff tendinitis. It is treated with NSAIDs and/or intra-bursal or intra-articular corticosteroids. The calcification tends to resolve when the symptoms resolve. If it occurs in a patient with significant renal failure, one should check for hyperphosphatemia, since this may precipitate hydroxyapatite formation in soft tissues. Shoulder exercises should be also used, especially when the pain improves.

Biceps tendinitis

Other than in acute injury, biceps tendinitis often accompanies other shoulder disorders such as impingement syndrome and rotator cuff tendinitis. Pain is felt over the anterior shoulder, and worsens when carrying objects with the elbow flexed.

Rupture of the biceps tendon (short head) may produce a prominent swelling of the belly of the muscle in the lower arm. Therapy includes rest from aggravating activities, maintenance of shoulder range of motion, NSAIDs, and occasionally corticosteroid injection into the biceps tendon sheath that runs through the bicipital groove. If the patient has impingement syndrome, injection into the subacromial bursa often also improves biceps tendinitis because of a communication with the biceps sheath.

Adhesive capsulitis (frozen shoulder)

Adhesive capsulitis (also referred to as frozen shoulder or periarthritis of the shoulder) is in part an inflammatory disorder that produces fibrosis and adhesions of the joint capsule leading to contracture of the capsule and limitation of range of motion of the joint. It may occur at other joints, but is most common in the shoulder. It may follow (by weeks or months) trauma or other illness that causes immobilization, such as myocardial infarction, pneumonia, major surgery, etc.

It occurs more often in women, particularly over the age of 50 years. One or both shoulders may be involved with an insidious onset of pain, stiffness, restriction of motion, and nocturnal pain. Examination will show more diffuse shoulder tenderness and restriction of both passive and active range of motion in most directions. External rotation will be the most restricted. If presenting after several months of symptoms, there may be very little motion (frozen shoulder).

Radiographs will be normal except perhaps showing osteopenia due to disuse. An arthrogram will confirm the contracture of the capsule, but is not often necessary for diagnosis.

Prevention is in the early mobilization of all patients recovering from illness or surgery. Otherwise, therapy includes a combination of physiotherapy gradually to improve range of motion, and NSAIDs or intra-articular corticosteroids to control pain. Failing this, surgical manipulation under general anesthesia has been used, but with small risks of inadvertent humeral fracture and soft tissue damage.

Patients may develop reflex sympathetic dystrophy in the hand of the affected side (this should present with diffuse hand swelling). See the topic Reflex sympathetic dystrophy for the diagnosis and treatment of this condition (page 175).

In the elderly, the differential diagnosis is polymyalgia rheumatica which may have similar symptoms, but in polymyalgia rheumatica there is also lower back and thigh pain and stiffness, which is not seen in simple adhesive capsulitis of the shoulder.

Acromioclavicular and sternoclavicular arthritis

Pain at these joints occurs in acute shoulder injuries, rheumatoid arthritis, osteoarthritis, seronegative spondyloarthropathies, crystal arthropathies, and septic arthritis. Septic arthritis at these sites is associated with intravenous (IV) drug use, with *Staphylococcus aureus* being the most common organism. Arthritis of these joints may coexist with other inflammatory causes of shoulder pain, and one may have to inject local anesthesia at these sites to determine its significance in the patient's complaint of shoulder pain.

Examination will reveal tenderness over the joint. In acromioclavicular arthritis there will be pain upon active abduction beyond 90°, increasing with further abduction and arm elevation (as opposed to impingement syndrome where there is a painful arc of abduction between 60° and 120° that improves if the arm is elevated beyond 120°). In sternoclavicular arthritis, most shoulder movements cause pain. Therapy includes NSAIDs, maintenance of shoulder range of motion, avoidance of activities that cause the pain, and occasionally intra-articular corticosteroids.

Glenohumeral arthritis

This is a much less common cause of shoulder pain than tendinitis. It occurs in patients with rheumatoid arthritis, osteoarthritis, and crystal arthropathy. In patients with these diseases, there may be coexistent shoulder tendinitis. A clue to glenohumeral arthritis is pain with internal rotation (the other cause of pain during internal rotation being adhesive capsulitis).

The treatment is aimed at the primary disease, but otherwise NSAIDs and occasionally intra-articular corticosteroids. One must also encourage physiotherapy to help maintain the rotator cuff that may suffer disuse atrophy.

See Appendix 2 for a table of shoulder and other regional disorders.

Section 3 – Localized pain

Most cases of elbow pain are due to either tendinitis or chronic pain syndromes.

Algorithmic Approach

Patients with chronic pain syndromes will often present with elbow or forearm pain, and be given a diagnosis of arthritis. This incorrect diagnosis results from failing to ask the patient about pain location.

If the pain is localized to the elbow or forearm region, then we are traveling down the algorithm. If swelling is absent, then the patient must have one of: tendinitis; osteoarthritis; or SLE.

(Olecranon bursitis is an exception here, in that it usually produces obvious swelling. See discussion below.)

SLE is easily addressed by considering the diagnostic criteria. Such patients rarely complain of elbow pain in any case. Tendinitis and osteoarthritis will be diagnosed by the techniques of examination described below.

If swelling is documented, consider how many joints are involved. The patient complaining of pain in one elbow, according to the algorithm, must have one of: palindromic arthritis; crystal arthropathy; septic arthritis; or spondyloarthropathy (which rarely affects the elbow).

Refer to Section 4 for details of these diseases, but essentially one will use pattern of attacks (palindromic arthritis), joint aspiration (crystal arthropathy, septic arthritis), and diagnostic criteria (spondyloarthropathy).

If there is swelling in more than one joint (the elbow or elsewhere), then the patient must have one of: rheumatoid arthritis; SLE; spondyloarthropathy; or crystal arthropathy.

The first three are easily addressed by asking questions regarding, and examining for, the diagnostic criteria. (Do not order X-rays for the spondyloarthropathy unless the clinical criteria are evident.) Crystal arthropathy requires aspiration for diagnosis.

Examination of the elbow

Normal ranges of motion are:

Flexion	160°
Extension	Fully straight

The examination proceeds as follows:

1. Begin by asking the patient to indicate the location of pain. Epicondylitis (tennis or golfer's elbow) may produce pain in the proximal forearm, whereas arthritis usually produces pain closer to the joint.

2. Observe for swelling. This may be on the posterolateral aspect of the elbow joint (ulnahumeral) or over the radiohumeral joint. (The joint formed by the olecranon process of the ulna and the humerus is described here as the elbow joint, whereas the radiohumeral joint is considered separately.) Swelling may also be due to olecranon bursitis, located over the posterior 'bend' or apex of the elbow (*Figure 3.10*). Compare one elbow with the other to detect swelling.

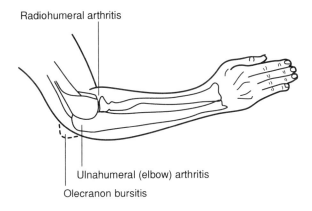

Fig. 3.10   Location of swelling in elbow disorders.

3. Observe for erythema, which suggests septic arthritis (or septic bursitis) or crystal arthropathy (or bursal involvement), and which mandates aspiration.

4. Have the patient flex and extend the elbow, and pronate and supinate the hand. Restriction of movement is almost always due to joint disorder, and one would therefore find that both passive and active motion were restricted and painful.

5. Palpate over the elbow joint with your hand posterior to the elbow during flexion and extension. Crepitus may be felt if osteoarthritis is present. Crepitus may also be felt during supination and pronation of the hand while palpating over the radiohumeral joint (*Figure 3.11*).

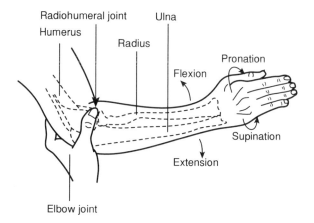

Fig. 3.11 Palpation for crepitus. Flex and extend as palm detects crepitus. Supinate and pronate as thumb detects crepitus.

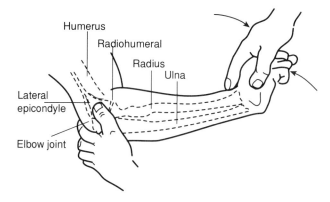

Fig. 3.12 Detecting lateral epicondylitis. Palpate the lateral epicondyle, while the patient makes a fist and extends wrist against resistance.

6. Use the maneuvers described below (and see *Figure 3.12*) to detect lateral epicondylitis (tennis elbow).

Key examination points

- Tennis elbow is the most common cause of elbow pain.
- Restricted elbow range of motion is due to arthritis.

The diagnosis and management of some specific elbow disorders is discussed below, emphasizing historical or physical features that aid in diagnosis. Physiotherapy exercises for elbow disorders are described in Appendix 1.

Olecranon bursitis

Olecranon bursitis may be due to crystal deposition or infection, and is common in rheumatoid arthritis. Some individuals, however, accumulate fluid in the bursa for no apparent reason. It produces a clearly visible swelling at the apex of the elbow (see *Figure 3.10*) and is often acutely painful, and sometimes erythematus. Pain may be referred along the ulnar border of the forearm.

The bursa should be aspirated to look for crystals or infection. NSAIDs may help crystal-induced bursitis, but intra-bursal corticosteroids are often more useful. Drainage of the asymptomatic bursal swelling is not often recommended as it tends to recur. Surgical excision may be helpful, but swelling and inflammation in the area may recur despite this. Infection should be surgically drained.

Tennis elbow (lateral epicondylitis)

Virtually all cases of elbow pain are tendinitis or chronic pain syndromes. Tennis elbow occurs in individuals whose activities include repeated gripping. This causes a complementary chronic strain of the wrist extensors. The patient complains of pain at the lateral arm which may radiate into the forearm, and weakness of grip. They may describe that specific activities such as lifting a pot (especially if it is heavy and requires a firm grip) brings on the pain as opposed to gripping a cup (which requires pinch activity more than the finger and wrist flexors).

The diagnosis can be confirmed by noting point tenderness at the attachment of the extensor muscles on the lateral humeral condyle (see *Figure 3.12*). Patients with chronic pain syndromes will often give a similar history, and have tenderness in this region (but also many other regions of the arm will be tender). One way of proving true tendinitis is that resisted wrist extension (particularly with a closed fist) is specifically painful. Your hand placed so as to tightly circumscribe the muscle bellies of the extensor muscles (about 10 cm below the elbow) will noticeably increase grip strength and lessen pain with grip, because it splints the muscle. Range of motion of the elbow should be normal.

For mild cases, avoidance of activities that worsen symptoms, use of a forearm 'wrap' or tensor band, and physiotherapy may suffice. The tensor band should be about 7.5–10 cm wide and should wrap around the forearm snugly starting about 2.5 cm below the elbow joint. Corticosteroid injections are also helpful.

Golfer's elbow (medial epicondylitis)

Golfer's elbow is much less common, but has a similar presentation to an overuse injury, affecting the wrist flexors. Point tenderness is found at the medial epicondyle, and worsened by resisted wrist flexion (particularly with a closed fist). One must consider ulnar nerve entrapment as a cause of the patient's symptoms, however, and examine the motor and sensory components of the nerve.

The treatment is as for tennis elbow, including physiotherapy.

Elbow and radiohumeral arthritis

Restriction of normal elbow range of movement or of normal supination and pronation of the hand virtually always indicates arthritis. The most common chronic form is secondary osteoarthritis in rheumatoid arthritis, while acute episodes are usually due to gout. The restriction that appears earliest in chronic arthritis is an inability to extend or straighten the arm.

In patients with osteoarthritis of the elbow, and particularly in those who may have shoulder and wrist arthritis that compromises upper limb function, surgical procedures to improve range of movement are helpful. It is also possible for flexion contractures to occur with chronic arthritis at this joint, which can be prevented by intensive physiotherapy exercises while the cause is being treated.

See Appendix 2 for a table of elbow and other regional disorders.

Section 3 – Localized pain

Painful hand or wrist

The diagnosis of the cause of hand or wrist pain is easily accomplished by a few questions and some specific examination techniques, as discussed below.

Algorithmic Approach

If a patient complains of hand or wrist pain, the first thing to consider is its localization. Patients with chronic pain syndromes will often present with hand or wrist pain, and indeed be given a diagnosis of hand arthritis. This incorrect diagnosis results from failing to ask the patient about pain localization and extent. Patients with chronic pain syndromes frequently have whole arm pain, but complain selectively (on one occasion) of hand pain alone.

If the pain is localized to the hand or wrist region, then we are traveling down the algorithm. If swelling is absent, then the patient must have one of: tendinitis/bursitis; osteoarthritis; or SLE.

SLE is addressed easily by considering the diagnostic criteria. Tendinitis and osteoarthritis will be diagnosed by the techniques of examination described below.

If the patient does complain of swelling, be sure that this has been observed by a physician, since patients with chronic pain syndromes may complain of swelling that is not really there. If swelling is documented, consider how many joints are involved. If only one joint, then the patient must have one of: palindromic arthritis; crystal arthropathy; septic arthritis; or spondyloarthropathy.

For details refer to each of the descriptions of these diseases in Section 4, but essentially one will use pattern of attacks (palindromic arthritis), joint aspiration (crystal arthropathy, septic arthritis), and diagnostic criteria (spondyloarthropathy).

If more than one joint in the hand and wrist (or joints elsewhere) are swollen then the patient must have one of: rheumatoid arthritis; SLE; spondyloarthropathy, or crystal arthropathy.

The first three are addressed easily by asking questions regarding, and examining for, the diagnostic criteria. (Do not order X-rays for the spondyloarthropathy unless the clinical criteria are evident.) Crystal arthropathy requires aspiration for diagnosis.

Examination of the hand and wrist

One must be able to distinguish clearly between tendinitis and synovitis, since they may each produce some pain and swelling over the region of a joint. To do this compare active and passive movement. When there is joint synovitis, movement is painful and limited in range equally when the joint is actively moved (the patient contracts a muscle to move the joint) or passively moved (the examiner flexes or extends the joint, with the patient's muscles relaxed). When a patient has tendinitis, however, there is considerably less pain and a better range of movement during passive testing (because the muscles and tendons are relaxed and you move the joint) than during active testing (when muscles and tendons are contracted by the patient).

For example, with wrist pain and swelling, ask the patient to extend and flex the wrist. Note the amount of movement possible. Now have the patient relax, and you slowly flex and extend the wrist. If the range you accomplish for the same degree of patient discomfort is the same as the patient could, they have joint synovitis. If the range you accomplish (passive) is greater than the patient can (active), then they have tendinitis. It is possible, such as in rheumatoid arthritis, to have both at the same time, but otherwise this is rare, and the differentiation should not be difficult. This method can be applied for most regions where one notes swelling and restriction of movement, and would like to determine whether arthritis (synovitis) is responsible, or simply tendinitis.

Normal ranges of motion are:

Wrist flexion	80–90°
Wrist extension	80–90°
MCP	90°
Interphalangeal flexion	90°
Metacarpal extension	Fully straight
Interphalangeal extension	Fully straight

The examination proceeds as follows:

1. Begin with having the patient indicate the site of pain. This can often lead to the diagnosis quite readily. If the pain is near the base of the thumb, for example, then the patient either has osteoarthritis of the carpometacarpal joint of the thumb or De Quervain's tendinitis (abductor pollicus longus and extensor pollicus brevis). If the pain is throughout the wrist then the patient either has osteoarthritis or one of the monoarticular arthropathies listed in the algorithmic approach above. Pain over the palm and /or flexor surfaces of the fingers indicates flexor tendinitis.

    Symptoms from arthritis involving the hand are usually very well localized to specific joints. If the proximal and distal interphalangeal joints are involved, osteoarthritis is likely. If the MCP with or without other hand joints are affected, then the other arthropathies in the algorithm are likely.

2. Next note any swelling, and determine whether it is bony swelling (hard) or not (soft). Bony swelling is seen at the proximal and distal interphalangeal joints in osteoarthritis (producing Bouchard's and Heberden's nodes, *Figure 3.13*). Then look for erythema. It indicates septic arthritis or crystal arthropathy until proven otherwise (which requires joint aspiration). Also look at the fingernails for pits which are a clue to psoriatic arthritis, as is psoriasis elsewhere.

3. Palpate for swelling and synovitis by detecting a softness or cushion lying between your finger tips and the bony margins of the joint. (Compare how easily you can palpate the bony margins of your hand joints to ones that have synovitis.) You should be able to feel the margins of the MCP joints, and a gap between them on the lateral and medial sides where the two bones come together to form a joint (*Figure 3.14*). For the proximal and

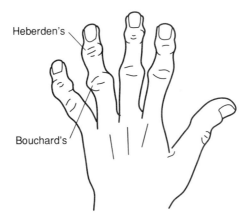

Heberden's

Bouchard's

Fig. 3.13 Bouchard's and Heberden's nodes in osteoarthritis of the hands.

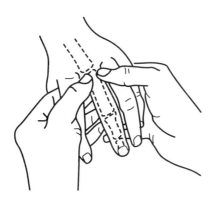

Fig. 3.14 Palpation of metacarpophalangeal joints for synovitis. The synovial tissue makes the distal end of the metacarpal bone and proximal end of the phalangeal bone more difficult to feel.

distal interphalangeal joints, place your forefinger and thumb on either side of the joint, and by gently squeezing the sides, you will notice that the thumb of your other hand, if lying on top of the joint, will feel as if it is being pushed up when you squeeze the sides of the joint. This indicates an effusion (*Figure 3.15*).

4. Then palpate for tenderness at the carpometacarpal joint (*Figure 3.16*) and perform Finkelstein's test (*Figure 3.17*) to diagnose either osteoarthritis of

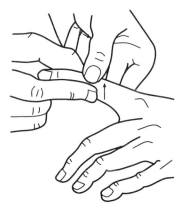

Fig. 3.15 Palpation of interphalangeal joints for synovitis. Bulging upward will be felt while pinching the medial and lateral aspects of the joint.

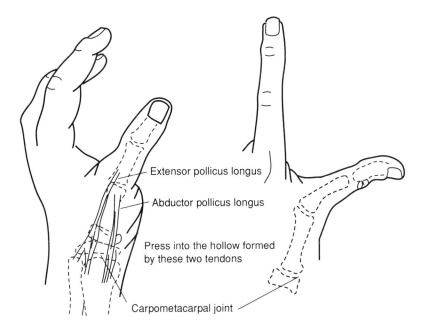

Extensor pollicus longus

Abductor pollicus longus

Press into the hollow formed by these two tendons

Carpometacarpal joint

Fig. 3.16 Palpation for tenderness in osteoarthritis of the carpometacarpal joint.

the carpometacarpal joint of the thumb or De Quervain's tendinitis. (See descriptions of these specific disorders below.)

5. Next compare passive and active range of movement. If there is a joint problem, the patient will have pain and restriction of movement regardless of whether they move their joint (active) or you move it for them (passive). Start with flexion and extension of the wrist and compare active and passive movements. (The latter can be done as shown in *Figure 3.18.*) Then test flexion of the metacarpophalangeal and interphalangeal joints (*Figures 3.19* and *3.20*).

Abductor and extensor pollicus brevis tendons

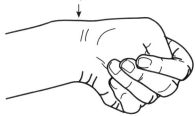

Fig. 3.17 Finkelstein's test.

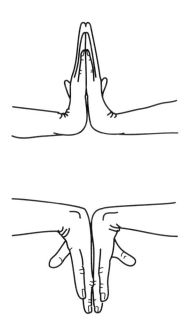

Fig. 3.18 One method of testing passive range of motion of the wrist.

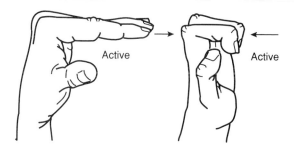

Fig. 3.19 Flexion of metacarpophalangeal joints.

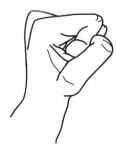

Fig. 3.20 Flexion of interphalangeal joints. (A simple screen of active flexion – making a fist.)

Flexor tendinitis limits the patient's attempts (active) to make a fist, but you will be able to close the hand for them (passive) if they are relaxed (*Figure 3.21*). If there is a difference between active and passive flexion, palpate the distal palm just before the origins of the fingers as you passively flex and extend the fingers. You will feel crepitus and perhaps nodules which result from chronic tendinitis (*Figure 3.22*).

Key examination points

- Passive range of motion better than active range indicates tendinitis.
- Equal restriction of range of active and passive motion indicates arthritis.
- Pain near the thumb or radial aspect of the wrist is either osteoarthritis of the thumb or De Quervain's tendinitis.

The diagnosis and management of some specific hand disorders is discussed below, emphasizing historical or physical features that aid in diagnosis. Physiotherapy exercises for hand disorders are described in Appendix 1.

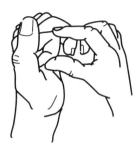

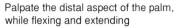

Palpate the distal aspect of the palm, while flexing and extending

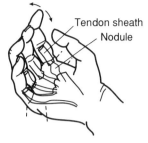

Tendon sheath
Nodule

Fig. 3.21 Passive flexion of metacarpo-phalangeal and interphalangeal joints.

Fig. 3.22 Palpation for flexor tendinitis and tendon nodules of the hands.

De Quervain's tendinitis

When a patient complains of pain near the base of the thumb, or radial aspect of the wrist, they usually have either osteoarthritis of the carpometacarpal joint of the thumb, or De Quervain's tendinitis (the abductor pollicus longus and extensor pollicus brevis located on the radial side of the wrist, attaching to the thumb). If one presses into the 'hollow' on the radial aspect of the wrist between the two prominent extensor and abductor tendons of the thumb (the anatomic 'snuff box') pain will be produced if osteoarthritis of the carpometacarpal joint exists (see *Figure 3.16*).

Examination in De Quervain's tendinitis will show tenderness over the radial styloid region. It is made worse by having the patient make a fist with the thumb inside, and then the examiner forcibly adducts the wrist (which pulls this tendon taut). This helps to distinguish it clearly from wrist synovitis, as well as the fact that there is usually no swelling in this form or tendinitis (see *Figure 3.17*).

Therapy for De Quervain's tenosynovitis involves avoiding activities which worsen symptoms, using a wrist splint during activity, NSAIDs, and occasionally corticosteroid injections into the tendon sheath.

Flexor or extensor tendinitis of hand

This condition is commonly seen in inflammatory arthritis. One must distinguish tendinitis in the hand from synovitis of the finger joints, since each may cause finger swelling. The aforementioned test of comparing active versus passive range of motion is useful, since tendinitis in the digits may mimic arthritis (see *Figures 3.18–3.20*).

Therapy includes avoiding the activity causing the condition, NSAIDs, physio-therapy, and possibly corticosteroid injection into the tendon sheath.

Trigger finger (stenosing tendinitis)

When a patient complains of pain over the palmar surface of the fingers, this is often either tendinitis or chronic pain syndromes. Restriction of active move-ment (inability to make a fist) is seen in flexor tendinitis, but not in chronic pain syndromes. The passive range of flexion will also be greater than the active range in tendinitis. Inflammation within the tendon sheath of the finger flexor muscles after chronic overuse may lead to fibrosis. It occurs most often at sites of the normally pre-existing fibrous rings of the tendon sheath, just proximal to the MCP joints. Chronic abrasion of the tendon then leads to a tendon nodule, which eventually may become large enough to be trapped by the fibrous tunnel, and not allow the finger to extend, thus producing a trigger finger (see *Figure 3.21*).

Therapy includes modifying activity (changing to activities that do not rely so much on grasping), NSAIDs, and corticosteroid injections into the fibrous tendon sheath. If this is ineffective, surgical transection of the sheath may be necessary.

See Appendix 2 for a table of hand and other regional disorders.

Section 3 – Localized pain

Algorithmic Approach

When a patient complains of 'hip pain', ask them to localize it, as they will often point to the lateral aspect of the upper thigh and pelvis, where the pain of trochanteric bursitis is felt, rather than point to the inguinal region where true hip joint pain is felt. One must also determine whether or not they have diffuse lower limb pain, since patients with chronic pain syndromes have pain in this region as well (but also in many other sites).

If the pain is localized to one region, and that region is the lateral aspect of the upper thigh and pelvis, then the patient quite probably has bursitis. This can be confirmed by physical examination and specific symptoms of trochanteric bursitis (see below).

If one is considering true hip joint disorders (examination will confirm a hip joint problem as described below), because one is not going to see joint swelling, the entire lower part of the algorithm is to be considered. The patient may have one of: tendinitis/bursitis; osteoarthritis; or SLE.

The examination technique described below will deal with the first two. SLE would only rarely present with hip joint pain (unless they were on systemic corticosteroids, in which case avascular necrosis may have occurred), but in any case would be easily ruled out by the diagnostic criteria.

Again, not being able to detect hip joint swelling, it is necessary to include the part of the algorithm with arthritis. If only the one joint is involved, then the patient must have one of: palindromic arthritis; crystal arthropathy; septic arthritis; or spondyloarthropathy.

Palindromic arthritis at this joint is rare, as is crystal arthritis. Septic arthritis is considered if the problem is acute, and usually the patient has great difficulty moving at that joint. If one is suspicious of septic arthritis, aspiration is necessary (usually guided by radiologic means). Spondyloarthropathy is considered through the diagnostic criteria.

If both hip joints (or other joints with swelling) are involved, then the patient must have one of: rheumatoid arthritis; SLE; spondyloarthropathy; or crystal arthropathy.

The first three are easily addressed by asking questions regarding, and examining for, the diagnostic criteria. (Do not order X-rays for the spondyloarthropathy unless the clinical criteria are evident.) Crystal arthropathy requires aspiration for diagnosis.

Examination of the hip

Normal ranges of motion are:

Flexion   120°
Abduction   60°
Adduction   30°
External rotation   45°
Internal rotation   30°

The examination proceeds as follows:

1. Examination begins with asking the patient to indicate the site of their pain.
    If they point to the upper lateral thigh and pelvis, then palpate the region
    over the greater femoral trochanter for the tenderness of trochanteric
    bursitis (*Figure 3.23* and *3.24*). You may also continue with hip joint exam-
    ination to confirm that it is normal, as would be expected in trochanteric
    bursitis.

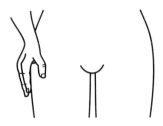

Fig. 3.23   The location of the pain of trochanteric bursitis.

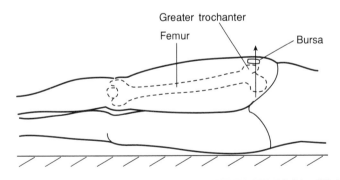

Fig. 3.24   Palpating over the trochanteric bursa. The bursa can be located in this position by tracing a perpendicular line from the medial aspect of the inguinal line to the
lateral thigh surface. The bony prominence of the trochanter is quite superficial.

2. Have the patient lie supine and test hip range of motion by first gently rolling the lower limbs, to test for pain (*Figure 3.25*). If the patient has significant pain in their hip with this gentle maneuver they are either malingering or have a serious problem (hip dislocation, hip septic arthritis).

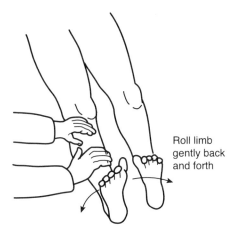

Roll limb
gently back
and forth

Fig. 3.25 Starting the hip joint examination.

Then ask the patient to flex their hip to the chest. At this point, a screening test for a normal hip joint is attempting to place the ankle of the limb being examined on the knee of the other limb, with the knee falling to the outside (making a figure four; *Figure 3.26*). If this can be accomplished, with no pain or restriction, the joint is normal.

If they cannot achieve full range or have pain with doing so, gently use passive range of testing to determine whether it is a joint or tendon disorder. A joint disorder will cause pain and restriction of movement regardless of whether it is active (the patient) or passive (you). If it is tendinitis/bursitis (such as psoas tendinitis or bursitis) then the patient will have normal hip flexion on passive testing.

3. Proceed with testing each motion, however, with the hip flexed at 90°, flex the knee to 90° and test internal and external hip rotation (*Figure 3.27*). Then test abduction and adduction. When testing abduction and adduction, the patient's pelvis must be kept stationary.

For abduction, place your left hand on the patient's left anterior iliac spine, and grasp their right ankle with your right hand. Pull their leg away from the midline toward you (*Figure 3.28*). Repeat on the other side (move to the other side of the examining table) by placing your right hand on the patient's right anterior iliac spine and grasping their left ankle with your left hand.

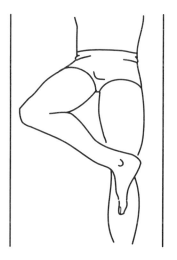

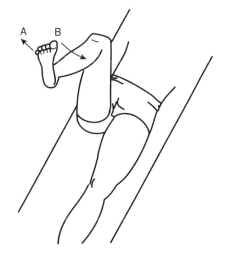

Fig. 3.26 Screening test for a normal hip joint.

Fig. 3.27 Testing hip internal and external rotation. (A = internal; B = external).

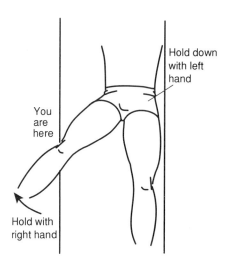

Hold down with left hand

You are here

Hold with right hand

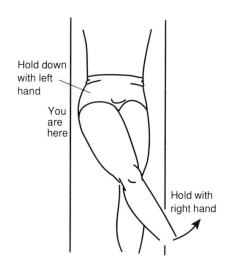

Hold down with left hand

You are here

Hold with right hand

Fig. 3.28 Testing hip abduction.

Fig. 3.29 Testing hip adduction.

For adduction, put your left hand on the patient's right anterior iliac spine, grasping their right ankle with your right hand. Lift the limb straight and high enough to clear the other limb as you bring it across and away from you (*Figure 3.29*). Repeat on the other side (move to other side of examining table), placing your right hand on the patient's left anterior iliac spine and grasping their left ankle with your left hand.

4. With the patient supine, and knowing whether or not they are capable of fully flexing their hip, ask them to place their hands behind the knee as they pull it towards their chest. Place your hand under their lumbar region to make sure they have flattened their spine, and look now at the other limb to see that you can easily make it flat against the bed while straight. If not, the patient has a hip contracture, and active physiotherapy is needed. Repeat on the other side (*Figure 3.30*).

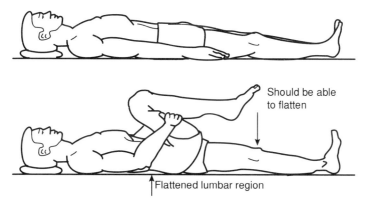

Should be able to flatten

Flattened lumbar region

Fig. 3.30 Detecting hip contractures.

5. You can test for limb length discrepancy by having the patient bend forward to reach for their toes when they are standing. Viewing from behind, you can observe the sacral promontory and if one side is higher, then that limb is longer (*Figure 3.31*). One can measure this with the patient supine, measuring each leg from the anterior iliac spine to the medial malleolus (*Figure 3.32*).

Key examination points

- Most 'hip pain' is actually trochanteric bursitis producing pain over the upper lateral thigh and pelvis.
- Making a 'figure four' is a good screen for hip joint disorder.

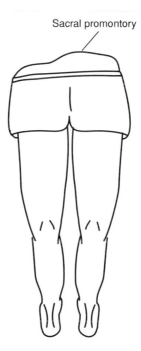

Fig. 3.31 Detecting limb length discrepancy. (Promontory higher on right. The right lower limb is longer than the left lower limb.)

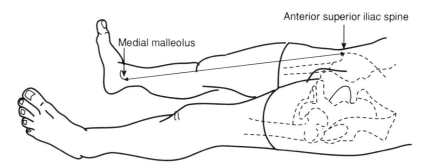

Fig. 3.32 Measuring lower limb length.

Trochanteric bursitis

When a patient complains that they have pain 'in the hip', but they actually point to the upper lateral thigh and pelvis, they almost always have trochanteric bursitis. This pain is often worse when lying on the affected side, often awakening the patient at night for this reason. They may also complain of pain with activity, however. True hip arthritis produces pain anteriorly, over the region of the inguinal ligament and below, sometimes referred to the knee region. Hip arthritis does not refer pain to the upper lateral thigh where the pain of trochanteric bursitis occurs.

Examination will reveal normal hip range of motion, and point tenderness when pressure is applied directly over the greater trochanter laterally.

NSAIDs may be helpful, but intra-bursal corticosteroids are also quite useful and often necessary.

See Appendix 2 for a table of hip and other regional disorders.

Section 3 – Localized pain

Painful knee

This section will deal with the nonorthopedic causes of knee pain, that is, pain that does not arise from primary abnormalities in the ligaments, and meniscal cartilage. In such cases, the patient gives a history of acute injury (usually sports injury). The knee pain arises from the medial or lateral collateral ligaments, the anterior or posterior cruciate ligaments, or the medial and lateral meniscal cartilage. These injuries produce a 'mechanical' disorder with pain during activity, knee locking, and 'giving-way' of the knee (which should make the patient fall). The reader is referred to a text of orthopedics or sports medicine for further information on the management of these injuries.

Algorithmic Approach

When a patient complains of knee pain, ask them to locate the pain and be certain that, although they are complaining of knee pain, it does not actually extend from their hips to their toes! Patients with chronic pain syndromes are sometimes told they have knee arthritis, when closer questioning reveals they have diffuse pain. If the patient complains of swelling, then this must be observed by a physician, because again patients with chronic pain syndromes may complain of knee swelling that actually is not there. Thus the patient with a knee disorder will complain of localized pain. If they complain of pain with no swelling, they must have one of: tendinitis/bursitis; osteoarthritis; or SLE.

(Osteoarthritis is listed in the algorithm with the diseases which cause localized pain and no swelling. For most joints, this is appropriate, but osteoarthritis of the knee may be associated with or without swelling.) Obviously, SLE can be ruled out by the diagnostic criteria. Thus, tendinitis/ bursitis or osteoarthritis remain, and the examination procedure below will describe how to diagnose these.

If the patient does describe knee swelling, then ask if there are any other joints involved with swelling. If not, then the patient must have one of palindromic arthritis; crystal arthropathy; septic arthritis; spondyloarthropathy; or knee osteoarthritis.

Refer to the details of these diseases (in Section 4), but essentially one will use pattern of attacks (palindromic arthritis), joint aspiration (crystal arthropathy, septic arthritis), and diagnostic criteria (spondyloarthropathy).

If there is more than one joint involved, then the patient must have one of: rheumatoid arthritis; SLE; spondyloarthropathy; crystal arthropathy; or bilateral knee osteoarthritis.

The first three are easily addressed by asking questions regarding, and examining for, the diagnostic criteria. (Do not order X-rays for the spondyloarthropathy unless the clinical criteria are evident.) Crystal arthropathy requires aspiration for diagnosis. After these steps have been taken, and are negative, bilateral knee osteoarthritis may be considered and confirmed by examination.

Examination of the knee

The examination technique described below will not allow the cause of knee pain to be determined in all patients, but will give a diagnosis in most cases. The more specific tests for ligament or meniscal pathology are not described here, as they are well delineated in orthopedic or sports medicine texts.

Normal ranges of motion are:

Flexion   140°
Extension   Fully straight

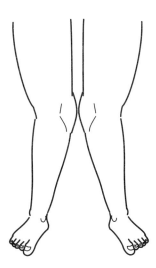

Fig. 3.33 Knee valgus.

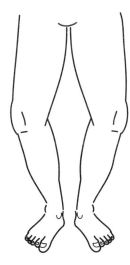

Fig. 3.34 Knee varus.

The examination proceeds as follows:

1. Begin with the patient standing if they can, and attempting to place their knees together. Look for valgus (knees touching and ankles not able to do so) and varus (ankles touching and knees not able to do so). These may be seen in osteoarthritis, which produces collateral ligament laxity, and isolated medial or lateral joint space narrowing (*Figures 3.33* and *3.34*).

2. View the posterior aspect of the knee while the patient is standing. This will make a Baker's cyst (bulging posteriorly of the joint capsule and synovium) visible. The normal appearance of the posterior knee and a Baker's cyst is shown in *Figure 3.35*. The standing position is the best for detecting this posterior bulging, since this position compresses the joint space and fluid is forced to areas of less constraint. It may also help to compare with the contralateral knee.

   With the patient still standing, note any flattening of the plantar arch, or signs of arch problems (including bunions, and hallux valgus). Some believe that knee pain is improved if patients who have arch collapse are given arch supports, and so it is worth trying.

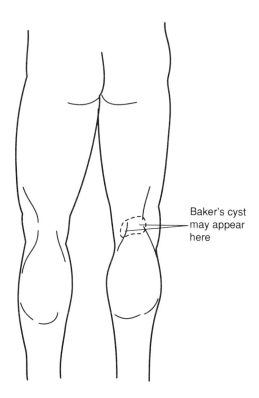

Fig. 3.35 Baker's cyst (posterior view of knee).

3. Have the patient lie supine, and ask them to indicate their site of pain. This simply allows one to be sure the patient's pain is localized to the knee region, again not extending down to their toes and up to their hips.

4. Note any erythema. If present, it is likely that the patient has a crystal arthropathy or septic arthritis, and joint aspiration is necessary.

5. Observe whether or not the knee appears swollen. If it does, there is obviously a joint problem. If not, look for evidence of swelling by the wipe test (or bulge sign) (*Figure 3.36*). This is performed by applying pressure with the hand over the suprapatellar bursa. The gap between your thumb and forefinger surrounds the proximal aspect of the patella, and your hand presses down gently on the thigh to force fluid into the lateral and medial compartments of the knee. Wipe the medial aspect of the knee gently from distal to proximal, close to the patella, and then wipe from proximal to distal along the lateral aspect of the knee close to the patella. As fluid that you initially pushed from medial to lateral is now pushed back by your hand, a bulge will appear over the medial aspect of the knee.

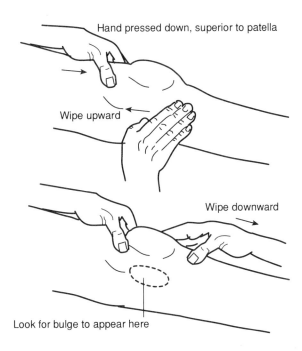

Fig. 3.36 Wipe test for knee effusion.

Before concluding that the wipe test is positive, be careful not to mistake moving superficial tissue (fat) for moving joint fluid. The wipe test produces a bulge on the medial aspect of the knee, at the midway point of the patella, not the 'jiggling' of fat generated by skin tension as you move your hands. It can be difficult in individuals with a lot of fat around the knee to be sure there is actually fluid there. One could examine the asymptomatic knee, and if you still produce what you believe is a positive test there (when it should not be positive) then probably you are just jiggling fat and not getting a positive wipe test (bulge sign) for fluid. An ultrasound of the knee can also detect effusions if you are having difficulty.

If the wipe test is negative, it means that either there is no effusion, or that the effusion is so large, one cannot move the fluid from side to side. To test for the latter, with your hand proximal to the patella as before, and the fingers of your other hand gently touching distal to the patella, pinch with the proximal fingers to move a fluid wave from proximal to distal (*Figure 3.37*).

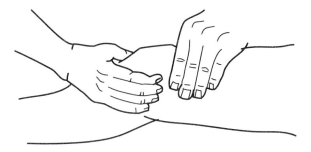

Fig. 3.37 Test for large knee effusion. 1. With upper hand, sudden pinch will move fluid inferiorly, towards lower hand. 2. With the lower hand gently gripping on either side of the inferior aspect to the patella, a bulge will push the fingers of your lower hand apart.

4. Palpate sequentially over the possible sites of inflamed bursae (*Figure 3.38*). First, note if there is a superficial small bulge (as if it is just under the skin) over the distal aspect of the patella. (This is pre-patellar bursitis.) Then press on the distal aspect of the patella. Tenderness here is patellar tendinitis. Next pinch with your thumb and forefinger around the lateral and medial aspects of the patellar tendon as if you are trying to get your thumb and forefinger to meet on the underside of the tendon. Tenderness here indicates infra-patellar bursitis which may coexist or be difficult to separate from patellar tendinitis. (The treatment is the same so it may not matter.) Finally, locate the site of the anserine bursa. With the knee extended, the anserine bursa is located three finger-breadths lateral to the tibial tuberosity. With the knee flexed to 90°, it is located three finger-breadths medial to the tibial tuberosity. Tenderness at this site is anserine bursitis, commonly coexisting with joint disorders and plantar arch collapse.

5. With the knee flexed to 90°, one can palpate the medial and lateral joint margins (tender in knee osteoarthritis and meniscal tears) (*Figure 3.39*).

6. Observe the patient actively flexing and extending their knee. As mentioned before, when a patient has limitation of active movement, test for range of passive movement (with the patient relaxed). If you can move the knee significantly further than the patient can, they have a tendinitis/bursitis. If you cannot accomplish much more than the patient then they have a joint problem. When you are passively flexing and extending the knee, place one hand over the entire anterior aspect of the knee. You will detect crepitus, seen in osteoarthritis and sometimes patellofemoral syndrome (*Figure 3.40*).

7. Test for laxity of the ligaments, comparing with the other knee as a control. Place both knees in 90° flexion. Look from the side to see if the normal prominence of the tibia is apparent. If not, it has slipped posteriorly due

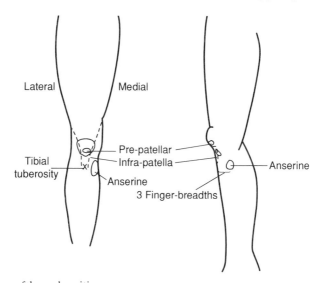

Fig. 3.38 Sites of knee bursitis.

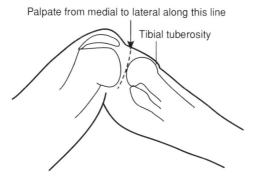

Fig. 3.39 Palpating knee joint margins.

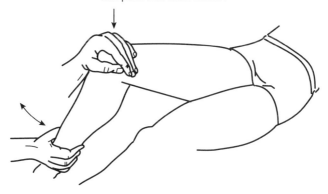

Fig. 3.40 Palpating for knee crepitus.

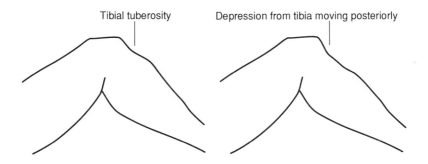

Fig. 3.41 Detecting posterior cruciate ligament laxity.

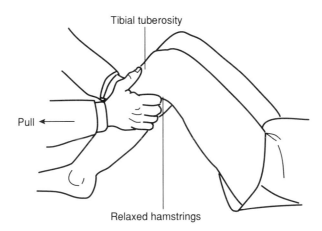

Fig. 3.42 Detecting anterior cruciate ligament laxity.

to posterior cruciate ligament laxity. With the knee in the 90° flexed position, place your forearm against the mid-tibia, and both hands around the upper calf with your fingers posteriorly. Make sure the hamstring muscles attached to the knee are not tense. Pull the calf forward with your hands while using your forearm to block movement of the body of the tibia. Look for the top of the tibia to protrude forward, indicating anterior cruciate laxity (see *Figures 3.41* and *3.42*).

Then, with the leg extended and relaxed, stress the lateral and medial collateral ligaments. These show laxity in osteoarthritis and injury (*Figure 3.43*).

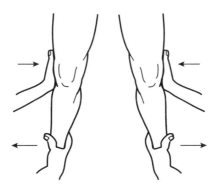

Fig. 3.43 Detecting medial and lateral collateral ligament laxity.

8. Patellofemoral syndrome remains a historical diagnosis rather than by physical examination. Tests for patellar irritability may not have the clinical significance that was once attached to them. With the knee extended and relaxed, place your fingers at the superior pole of the patella, and push the patella gently towards the feet. Now ask the patient to lift their leg straight and note pain or apprehension in the patient. This will cause pain under the patella in patellofemoral syndrome. It can be mildly painful to do this in normal subjects, however, so the pain must be significant. Have someone do the procedure on you, to know what it feels like. Another test sometimes used for this nebulous diagnosis of patellofemoral syndrome is to place pressure on the medial aspect of the patella, and push laterally as if you are trying to dislocate the patella. This will cause pain and apprehension in some patients with patellofemoral syndrome, but more so in those who are prone to patellar subluxation and dislocation (who have probably given a history of falling when this occurs) (*Figures 3.44* and *3.45*).

9. If you can find no source for the knee pain, immediately move to examination for the hip, since pain may be referred from the hip joint to the knee.

Treatment of various forms of knee arthritis is discussed elsewhere in the book. Anserine bursitis usually responds to hamstring stretches and arch supports if needed. Pre-patella and patella bursitis responds to NSAIDs or corticosteroid

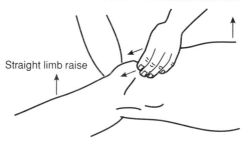

Fig. 3.44 Patellar irritability.

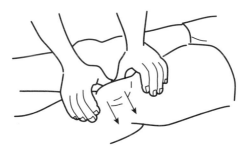

Fig. 3.45 Apprehension test.

injections. In the past, a lot of patients with patellofemoral syndrome were referred for arthroscopy and various surgical procedures, most of which have failed to benefit in the long term. Currently, it is recommended that the patient adopt a more conservative approach of exercises and patience. The patient must be told that it is up to them to do these exercises daily at home, and take on the responsibility for rehabilitation. They are not to become dependent on a physiotherapist.

If the patient does give a history of true locking (not just clicks or cracks, but an inability to straighten the knee once locked) or true patellar subluxation or dislocation, causing the patient to fall), then referral to an orthopedic surgeon is worthwhile.

Key examination points

- Valgus and varus are often signs of arthritis.
- Baker's cyst is detected by having the patient stand.
- A negative wipe test (or bulge sign) may mean that a large effusion is actually present.
- Palpate for each bursa, as bursitis is a common source of knee pain.
- Look for arch collapse.

See Appendix 2 for a table of knee and other regional disorders.

Section 3 – Localized pain

Painful foot or ankle

Algorithmic Approach

When a patient complains of pain about the ankle or foot, ask first about the distribution of pain. Some patients who complain of foot pain actually have whole lower limb pain, and a more appropriate series of questions will lead to the diagnosis of chronic pain syndrome. If, however, the pain is localized to one region, then one is traveling down the algorithm. If no swelling has been observed by a physician, the patient must have one of: tendinitis/bursitis (or arch collapse); osteoarthritis; or SLE.

SLE is addressed by the diagnostic criteria. The diagnosis of osteoarthritis or tendinitis/bursitis rests in the examination techniques described below.

If there is swelling present, then involvement of one joint means the patient has one of: palindromic arthritis; septic arthritis; crystal arthropathy; or spondyloarthropathy.

Refer to each of the chapters for these diseases, but essentially one will use pattern of attacks (palindromic arthritis), joint aspiration (crystal arthropathy, septic arthritis), and diagnostic criteria (spondyloarthropathy).

If the patient has more than one joint involved, then they must have one of: rheumatoid arthritis; SLE; spondyloarthropathy; or crystal arthropathy.

The first three are easily addressed by asking questions regarding, and examining for, the diagnostic criteria. (Do not order X-rays for the spondyloarthropathy unless the clinical criteria are evident.) Crystal arthropathy requires aspiration for diagnosis.

Examination of the foot and ankle

Specific tests for ligament laxity or joint instability are not discussed here, as they are well delineated in orthopedic or sports medicine texts. The joints to be examined are the ankle joint (which is made up of the tibiotalar joint and the talocalcaneal joint), the midfoot joints, the metatarsophalangeal joints, and the interphalangeal joints. Dorsiflexion is accomplished by anterior tibialis muscle chiefly, and plantar flexion by the gastrocnemius and soleus muscles which join to form the Achilles tendon.

Normal ranges of motion are:

Dorsiflexion (tibiotalar joint)	20°
Plantar flexion	45°
Supination or inversion (talocalcaneal joint)	30°
Pronation or eversion (talocalcaneal joint)	10°
Supination (midfoot)	20°
Metatarsophalangeal flexion	60°
Interphalangeal flexion	45°
Metatarsophalangeal extension	30°
Interphalangeal extension	Fully straight

The examination proceeds as follows:

1. Begin with the patient standing to note ankle valgus or varus and plantar arch collapse (may coexist). The ankle valgus or varus is best viewed from behind, with the patient's feet several centimeters apart. Note also hallux valgus and bunions which are signs that the patient needs arch supports and wider shoes (*Figures 3.46–3.49*).

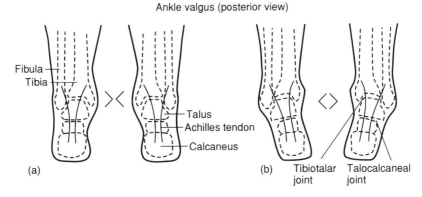

Ankle valgus (posterior view)

Fig. 3.46 (a) Ankle valgus posterior view and (b) ankle varus posterior view.

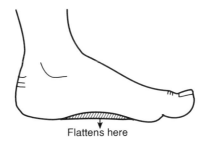

Flattens here

Fig. 3.47 The normal plantar arch and its collapse (medial view).

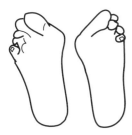 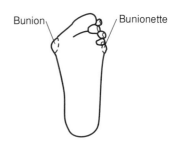

Fig. 3.48 Hallux valgus (commonly seen with plantar arch collapse).

Fig. 3.49 Bunions (1st toe) and bunionettes (5th toe).

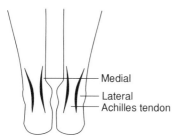 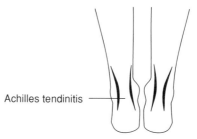

Fig. 3.50 The normal medial and lateral concavities between the Achilles tendon and the talus and calcaneus (posterior view).

2. Note any erythema. If present, this indicates either septic arthritis or crystal arthropathy, and aspiration is warranted.

3. Note swelling. Sometimes this is obvious. If not, ankle swelling can be detected by viewing it from posteriorly while the patient is standing. The Achilles tendon and calcaneous form two concavities medial and lateral from this view. If these concavities are filled, particularly when compared with the opposite ankle, then ankle joint swelling is probably present (*Figure 3.50*).

    It may be difficult to distinguish this from Achilles tendinitis with swelling, so one should then test active versus passive range of motion (see point 4). Achilles tendinitis will produce restriction of active plantar flexion (especially against resistance), but not passive plantar flexion, whereas joint synovitis will produce limitation in both active and passive movements.

    With the patient supine, swelling in the toes may be detected in the same manner as for the hand joints, palpating for the bony margins (synovitis makes them less easily felt) and squeezing the interphalangeal joints with forefinger and thumb on either side, while palpating for upward displacement of the thumb of your other hand as it rests on the joint. One can then compress the metatarsal joints as described below for the diagnosis of Morton's neuroma or synovitis (*Figures 3.51* and *3.52*).

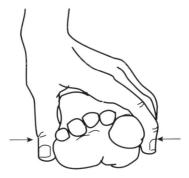

Fig. 3.51 Compression of the metatarsophalangeal joint.

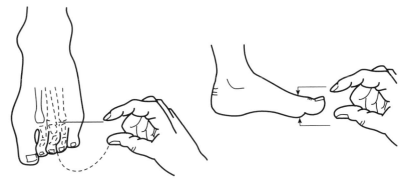

Fig. 3.52 Locating tenderness in Morton's neuroma.

4. Test active range of motion of each joint, and as one proceeds, if there is limitation or pain, test the passive range of that same joint.

    First begin with the tibiotalar joint (the joint at which dorsiflexion and plantar flexion occurs). Ask the patient to dorsiflex and plantar flex. Then test this range passively if it is restricted or painful (*Figure 3.53*).

    Second, test the second part of the ankle joint; the talocalcaneal joint. Place the ankle in dorsiflexion and hold it there. Then ask the patient to supinate and pronate the foot (*Figure 3.54*). To test this joint passively, continue to hold the foot in dorsiflexion and produce supination (inversion) and pronation (eversion) by moving the heel medial and lateral.

    Third, test the range of supination and pronation of the midfoot by eliminating any contribution from the ankle (hold the patient's ankle in dorsiflexion and cup the heel with one hand so that it cannot move laterally or medially. When this is done, grasp the midfoot and supinate (invert) and pronate (evert) (*Figure 3.55*).

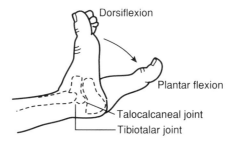

Fig. 3.53 Dorsiflexion and plantar flexion. (The tibiotalar joint is chiefly involved.)

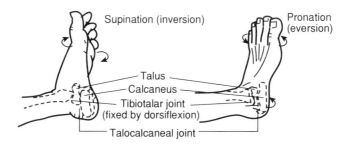

Fig. 3.54 Testing range of motion of the talocalcaneal joint.

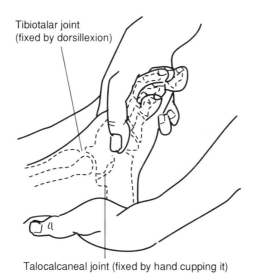

Fig. 3.55 Testing range of motion of the midfoot joints.

Finally, test active flexion and extension of the toes followed by passive testing if needed.

Again, if the active range of motion is limited or painful, check passive range of motion. If the patient has a joint problem, there will be pain and restriction whether the patient moves it (active) or you do (passive). If the passive range is better, then tendinitis/bursitis exists.

5. Palpate the region between the Achilles tendon and the calcaneous by pinching with your forefinger on one side and your thumb on the other (*Figure 3.56*). Tenderness here is due to retrocalcaneal bursitis, often present with Achilles tendinitis.

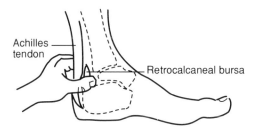

Fig. 3.56   Palpating for retrocalcaneal bursitis (medial view).

6. Palpate the base of the heel for tenderness seen in plantar fasciitis and arch collapse.

Key examination points

- Plantar arch collapse is the most common cause of ankle and foot pain.
- Arch collapse may play a role in knee pain.

The diagnosis and management of some specific foot and ankle disorders is discussed below, emphasizing again historical or physical features that aid in diagnosis. Physiotherapy exercises for ankle disorders are described in Appendix 1.

Plantar arch collapse

Whenever a patient complains of pain in the toes, ankle, anterior tibial region, or knee, examine the plantar arch. If it is flattened, this is often an explanation for or a contributing factor to the patient's symptoms. Patients with these complaints seldom have arthritis as the cause, and do not need any therapy other than arch supports.

Collapse of the plantar arch (longitudinal and transverse) occurs over many years in most cases, and eventually leads to symptoms of heel pain, pain under the toes, pain over the dorsum of the foot, ankle pain, anterior tibial pain, and even knee pain. The pain is usually worse with walking, or at the end of the day, especially if the individual has spent a lot of time standing or walking on a hard surface. If one cannot find obvious swelling in these joints, then this mechanical factor should be considered.

Patients with significant foot pain should get custom fitted arch supports. While arch supports can be expensive, they actually save the health care system money when compared with the high cost of repeated physician visits, NSAIDs, and physiotherapy. Some believe that patients with mechanical back pain may even benefit from arch supports. The best test is to try them. It is common for patients, even those without plantar fasciitis, to complain of discomfort when wearing arch supports. This discomfort is a result of a proper arch support now pushing upward on the sole. Have the patient wear their arch supports for only 1–2 hours a day initially, to adjust slowly to the support. They should try to lengthen the time they spend in the shoes with arch supports, and in a few weeks can usually wear them without difficulty.

Plantar fasciitis

If a patient complains of pain under the heel, particularly when they first start walking (i.e. upon awakening), consider plantar fasciitis.

Inflammation at the site of attachment of the plantar fascia to the calcaneous occurs following repeated trauma (walking, running) or as part of a seronegative spondyloarthropathy. Pain is worst on weight bearing and may spread to involve the entire sole. Examination may reveal collapse of the longitudinal arch on walking (as a predisposing factor) and tenderness over the center of the heel. One does not require an X-ray to demonstrate a 'bone spur' at the site since this is irrelevant. (Bone spurs are a result of plantar fasciitis, not the cause.) The condition may occur in the absence of such a spur and these spurs may exist in normal subjects.

Therapy includes either heel cups/supports or complete arch supports, and occasionally corticosteroid injections at the most tender site over the calcaneus. Arch supports may not be tolerated when the condition remains painful, but should be introduced as soon as tolerable.

March fracture (stress or fatigue fracture)

If a patient develops sudden onset of pain and swelling over the dorsum of the foot, they either have gout or a march fracture. March fracture should also be suspected in the patient with foot pain that has not responded to arch supports.

March fracture usually occurs in women, especially if they have been walking or jogging for longer or more strenuous periods than usual. It will produce pain and swelling over the forefoot, and may be quite acute so that it mimics gout, but since gout is distinctly uncommon in women (especially if they are not on diuretics and do not have renal disease), one should consider a march fracture instead. Other than this fracture or gout, there are only rare conditions which could produce forefoot swelling. Occasionally, there may be bruising associated with the swelling, and this is not seen in gout. Also, gout attacks subside in less than a week. The diagnosis can be made 3–6 weeks later, by seeing a nondisplaced fracture healing with callus, usually of the third metatarsal shaft. Bone scans will also detect such fractures early. Many cases resolve spontaneously over days to weeks, but one may also consider the use of arch supports and a tensor band or elastoplast around the forefoot, as well as NSAIDs. If the fracture is displaced, or fails to improve after a few weeks, then an orthopedic surgeon should see the patient and casting be used.

Morton's neuroma

When a patient complains of pain in the toes or under the toes, consider either plantar arch collapse (prescribe an arch support if so), arthritis (look for actual swelling and restriction of movement at the MTP joints, or evidence of arthritis in other joints), or a Morton's neuroma.

Entrapment of interdigital nerves between the metatarsal heads (and possibly a ganglion in the region) will produce sudden, sharp pains 'in the toes'. (This condition is sometimes referred to as acute inflammation of anterior metatarsal heads.)

Examination will reveal normal MTP joint range of motion with no swelling, and exquisite tenderness on palpation in the interdigital space involved. That is, the pain will be worst when one pinches between the toes rather than right over the MTP joints. Compression of the metatarsal heads by gripping the foot may reproduce the symptoms (see *Figures 3.51* and *3.52*). Treatment consists of wearing wider shoes, avoiding high-heels, cushioning orthotics for the metatarsal heads, arch supports if needed, and occasionally corticosteroid injection between the metatarsal heads where the pain is reproduced. Surgical excision of the neuroma is considered if all else fails.

Flexor or extensor tendinitis of the ankle

This condition is commonly seen in inflammatory arthritis, or as an overuse injury. One must distinguish tendinitis from synovitis of the ankle and foot joints. The aforementioned test of comparing active versus passive range of motion is useful (test dorsiflexion and plantar flexion passively and actively).

Achilles tendinitis is the most common, and is diagnosed by demonstrated pain or restriction of motion during active plantar flexion (especially against resistance), which is not present during passive plantar flexion. Retrocalcaneal bursitis may occur with Achilles tendinitis or on its own, but treatment is not any different.

Similarly, tendinitis of the anterior muscles will be demonstrated by finding pain or restriction of motion during active dorsiflexion (especially against resistance) that is not present during passive dorsiflexion.

Therapy includes avoiding the activity causing the overuse, NSAIDs, arch supports if needed, and physiotherapy exercises. Corticosteroid injections for foot or ankle tendinitis are not often used because of the concern that tendon rupture may occur (especially of the Achilles tendon).

Anterior leg pain

While anterior leg pain may arise from either 'shin splints' (thought to involve periostitis of the tibia, occurring as an overuse injury, or in active individuals with plantar arch collapse) or anterior leg muscles (e.g. tibialis anticus tendinitis), it is also very common in chronic pain syndromes. Make sure, therefore, that you have asked the patient about pain localization and whether or not they have pain in other sites on the lower limb.

Shin splints or tendinitis are diagnosed by demonstrating more pain and restriction of active dorsiflexion (especially against resistance) than passive dorsiflexion. The treatment for 'shin splints' or anterior tendinitis is reduced activity, physiotherapy exercises, and prescription of arch supports if needed.

See Appendix 2 for a table of foot and other regional disorders.

Section 3 – Localized pain

Osteoarthritis

In examining the patient with localized pain as demonstrated in the preceding sections, an arthritic disorder may have been diagnosed. Osteoarthritis is the most common form of arthritis in most joints, although in many cases it is the result of some other form of chronic arthritis (like rheumatoid arthritis). These other forms of arthritis would have been distinguished by the presence of joint swelling and gradual evolution into osteoarthritis as a complication. Whatever the cause, this section will discuss what to do with the diagnosis of osteoarthritis.

Algorithmic Approach

The algorithm suggests osteoarthritis does not cause swelling. It may in a few cases, especially the knee. The important use of the algorithm here is that the pain will be localized, and therefore one must be careful not to give a patient with fibromyalgia such a diagnosis. Careful questioning on the pain location and distribution will prevent this.

Osteoarthritis, then, is considered when there is localized pain with no swelling in the hands or wrists. (The other possibilities in the algorithm being tendinitis/bursitis, or SLE.)

It is considered in knee pain with no swelling. (The other possibilities in the algorithm being tendinitis/bursitis, or SLE.)

It is considered in hip pain (true hip joint pain as described below), and shoulder pain with no observable swelling. (The other possibilities in the algorithm being tendinitis/bursitis, or SLE.)

Lastly, it is considered in knee pain with swelling, but then so too must rheumatoid arthritis, SLE, spondyloarthropathy, and crystal arthropathy.

Osteoarthritis is thought by some to be a disease of cartilage with secondary bone changes. It is characterized chiefly by cartilage loss and a hypertrophic bone response around the joint. While in the past inflammation was not considered to be an important feature, it clearly does play a role in symptoms, and may be involved in cartilage destruction.

Osteoarthritis has a wide spectrum of clinical features ranging from radiographic and pathologic evidence of disease without symptoms to severe symptomatic and destructive disease. It is thought to occur most commonly as a result of abnormal physical forces that cause damage to normal articular cartilage, via repeated microtrauma from these forces. The cartilage is unable to repair proteoglycan loss, which then alters the cartilage matrix in structure. A simultaneous or subsequent cascade of enzymatic activity causes further degradation of the cartilage. Secondary to these events, release of cartilaginous breakdown products stimulate the synovium, and synovitis (usually mild) occurs. There is much debate about the exact mechanisms of what is a complex, chronic process, and the above is a simplified description. There are also some metabolic diseases which lead to inadequate cartilage function, that cannot cope with normal articular stresses, as in ochronosis, for example.

Whenever a patient is found to have osteoarthritis, one should always ask why it has occurred because there may be some factors that can be addressed and changed. See *Table 3.1* for a classification of osteoarthritis, recognizing that this classification is still evolving.

Table 3.1   Classification of osteoarthritis according to pathogenesis

Chronic abnormal forces on normal cartilage
Fractures healing with malalignment
Fracture nonunion
Obesity
Leg length discrepancy
Previous ligament tears and instability
Neuropathic (Charcot) joints
     diabetic neuropathy
     syphilis
     leprosy
     syringomyelia and other sensory neuropathies
Spinal apophyseal (facet) and intervertebral joints

Direct damage to cartilage
Inflammation
     rheumatoid arthritis
     crystal arthropathy
     septic arthritis
Fractures with intra-articular component
Direct trauma to cartilage (e.g. recurrent dislocations)
Loose bodies
(?) Repeated intra-articular corticosteroids

Abnormal cartilage
Metabolic diseases
     hemochromatosis
     ochronosis
     Wilson's disease
     acromegaly
     hyperparathyroidism
Epiphyseal dysplasia
Genetic disorders of collagen
Diffuse idiopathic skeletal hyperostosis
Aging process

Patients with chronic pain syndromes are sometimes told they have osteoarthritis as a cause for their joint pain (even though the patient is 35 years old!). Learn to recognize the findings of chronic pain syndromes, and make the proper diagnosis, sparing the patient worry about 'degenerative' arthritis.

Clinical manifestations

As previously stated, the correlation between radiographic changes and symptoms is variable. The best correlation is in the knee and hip. The most common symptom is pain, worsened by activity, improved by rest, and associated with mild, if any, joint swelling (except in the knee where swelling may be prominent). Morning stiffness is usually of less than 15 minutes duration. The patient may eventually develop pain at rest (poor prognosis), nocturnal pain (poor prognosis), and progressive loss of joint motion due to pain, large osteophytes impeding the range, joint contracture, and in some cases, ankylosis. Any synovial joint may be involved, but the DIP and PIP joints of the hand, the trapeziometacarpal joint of the thumb, spine joints, hips, and knees are the most common. Examination may reveal bony enlargement, deformity, ligamentous instability, synovitis, crepitus with range of motion, and decreased range of motion.

Patients with generalized osteoarthritis tend to be middle-aged women, with polyarticular hand involvement, Heberden's and Bouchard's nodes (cartilaginous and bony enlargement at the DIP and PIP joints, respectively), knee, spine, and hip involvement, positive family history, and overall good functional outcome.

Erosive, inflammatory osteoarthritis is a much less common form involving the interphalangeal hand joints with marked synovitis, subchondral erosions and joint destruction, with deformity and ankylosis. It tends not to involve other joints and may be confused with other inflammatory forms of arthritis (e.g. rheumatoid arthritis).

Isolated involvement of the hip, knee, and spine joints is also common, especially when there are underlying factors such as childhood bone deformities, avascular necrosis, trauma, and obesity. In the knee, medial and patellofemoral compartment involvement are the most common, although the lateral compartment may be involved. Both hip and knee involvement are often unilateral only, and if the patient has not developed contralateral involvement within 4 years of involving the one joint, it is likely to occur later in only 10%. Hip disease is often complicated by low back pain (due to compensatory lordosis, although apophyseal joint involvement may also exist).

Hip osteoarthritis tends to produce pain in either the inguinal region, medial thigh, or referred to the buttocks and the knee. When a patient gestures that their pain is located over the upper lateral aspect of the thigh and pelvis, this is likely to be trochanteric bursitis rather than hip osteoarthritis. Patients do not realise that hip joint pain is felt anteriorly or referred to the knee. The lateral aspect of the upper thigh and pelvis is not the hip joint. Further, if a patient has full abduction and rotation of the hip, then hip arthritis is unlikely to be responsible for the patient's pain.

Spine involvement occurs at the fibrocartilaginous joints articulating with the intervertebral discs and at the apophyseal (facet) joints. The term degenerative disc disease or spondylosis is usually used for the former. The disc narrowing may cause subluxation of posterior apophyseal joints, and anterior vertebral bone spurs are produced as well. The vertebrae most often involved are C5, T8, L3, and L4. Spondylolisthesis (forward translation of one vertebra upon the one below) may occur. There is little relationship between the degree of radiological abnormalities of the spine and back pain. Some patients have back pain with normal X-rays, and terrible X-ray changes with no symptoms. See the sections on the painful back and the painful neck, pages 146 and 156.

A condition which may be related to osteoarthritis is diffuse idiopathic skeletal hyperostosis (DISH), characterized by ossification along the ligaments of the anterior and lateral spine, appearing to bridge large spurs from adjacent vertebrae. The process is usually symmetrical and may involve all regions of the spine. Ossification occurs at other sites of entheses (tendon insertions) such as the plantar fascia insertion. Affected patients may have some restriction of spine motion. It is differentiated from ankylosing spondylitis by absence of sacroiliac involvement, and by the much greater degree of ossification in DISH. Such ossification does occur in other forms of osteoarthritis of the spine but to a lesser degree, with asymmetry.

Chondromalacia patellae (patellofemoral, or anterior knee compartment syndrome) is thought to result from abnormal forces due to recurrent lateral patellar subluxation, and may be a form of osteoarthritis. Certain 'tracking forces' are responsible for keeping the patella in the intercondylar groove during knee flexion and extension. Knee valgus, deficiency of the vastus medialis muscle, shallow intercondylar groove, and possible plantar arch collapse or ankle valgus (in older patients) may predispose to this condition. Patients are usually women, and complain of pain during climbing (or sometimes descending) stairs, any activity which requires significant knee flexion, or prolonged stationary knee flexion. Patellofemoral syndrome is a more general term that reminds us that we do not always know the pathophysiology involved (i.e. chondromalacia patella in a young teenager is not equivalent to osteoarthritis in an older patient, since chondromalacia patella tends to resolve as they grow older). One must be cautious, furthermore, in labeling a patient with osteoarthritis, since many cases of patellofemoral syndrome are of unknown cause and have a much better prognosis than most patients will understand osteoarthritis to have. Patients with chronic pain syndromes are often under the belief that they now have some form of chronic osteoarthritis of the knee.

The treatment is strengthening exercises to improve vastus medialis forces (see Appendix 1), knee wraps or sleeves, or in some cases, surgery if conservative therapy fails. The latter should be considered in only cases of documented patellar dislocation (which would have caused episodes of knee pain with falling in most cases), since the many patients who have in the past received a number of procedures for knee pain have had a poor long-term outcome. Surgery for pain is often less than optimal in its results.

Laboratory findings

Typically, osteoarthritis is not associated with hematologic abnormalities, or elevation of the ESR. One should consider the secondary causes of osteoarthritis such as Wilson's disease, hemochromatosis (especially when MCP joints involved), etc. and pursue appropriate investigations for these diseases.

Radiographs are key to the diagnosis, showing joint space narrowing from loss of articular cartilage, bone sclerosis, osteophytes, and occasionally subchondral cysts in the peri-articular bone. In severe cases, loose bodies, subluxation and other deformities may occur. Ankylosis (the union of the bones of a joint) is sometimes seen in erosive inflammatory osteoarthritis. Weight-bearing radiographs should be used for the lower limb joints in order that the two opposing articular surfaces are in contact. Any loss of cartilage will be demonstrated as joint narrowing, which may not be apparent in the nonweight-bearing position because the joint surfaces are distracted. Osteoarthritis may affect the sacroiliac joints, as judged by radiology, but whether or not this is symptomatic is unclear.

Synovial fluid appears grossly normal with normal viscosity, and < 3000 white blood cells (WBC)/mm^3. The exceptions are erosive, inflammatory osteoarthritis and in the presence of crystal-induced inflammation. Calcium pyrophosphate (pseudogout), uric acid (gout), and calcium hydroxyapatite crystals are commonly found in osteoarthritic joints and may be responsible for inflammatory episodes in some patients, although they may also be found in asymptomatic individuals. The crystals may be involved in the pathogenesis of osteoarthritis in these patients.

Treatment

Since pain is the most significant symptom, treatment with analgesics is important. Acetaminophen (paracetamol), particularly when used on a more regular basis during symptomatic periods, may be effective alone. NSAIDs are of benefit likely because of their analgesic effect, and also because of their anti-inflammatory effect, particularly in erosive, inflammatory osteoarthritis. NSAIDs may have a role in the prevention of cartilage destruction, but this is not yet known. Studies which document (perhaps by MRI) the effects of NSAIDs on the natural history of cartilage destruction are needed. It also remains controversial as to whether or not some NSAIDs may actually be detrimental, but their widespread use does not seem to be associated with a clinical worsening. Acetaminophen (paracetamol) is less expensive and associated with fewer adverse effects than NSAIDs. For knee osteoarthritis, it is as effective as NSIADs. On the other hand, the degree of inflammation in some patients requires an NSAID for effective symptom relief. Patients may benefit from prophylactic use (such as 1 hour prior to activity) of either type of drug.

There may be benefit to reducing adverse mechanical forces. Weight loss in obesity, use of a cane (placed on the 'good' side to redistribute body weight away from the affected knee), correction of leg length discrepancy, and improving supporting muscle strength may be helpful. Intra-articular corticosteroid injections are useful in some patients, although there is a concern that frequent injections (> 3 per year) may accelerate osteoarthritis.

Agents thought to actually protect or encourage repair of the cartilage are being considered and used. These include glucosaminoglycan compounds, metalloproteinase inhibitors, hyaluronate, and collagen. Numerous studies are currently evaluating their benefit. Surgical lavage of the joint has not been of proven benefit, although removing possibly symptomatic loose bodies may help.

Quadriceps strengthening and hamstring stretching exercises may be useful in maintaining the supportive benefit of the muscles.

Custom-made braces and insoles are sometimes helpful in reducing loads on the affected knee compartment, reducing pain and improving function.

Joint replacement is most successful in the knee or hip joints, there being far fewer successes with other sites. Indications for joint replacement depend on the patient's desired and achievable level of activity. Pain at rest, marked limitation in walking distance (i.e. less than one block), and persistent significant symptoms despite conservative therapy are indications. One must realize that joint prosthetic lifetimes are 10–15 years in hip replacement and 5–10 years in knee replacement, so that replacement in young patients may be complicated by eventual need for a second prosthesis. Tibial osteotomies that alter varus or valgus forces at the knee may be a temporizing measure prior to joint replacement in younger patients.

DOs and DON'Ts of osteoarthritis

DO consider use of regular acetaminophen (paracetamol) in the elderly instead of NSAIDs for osteoarthritis, since some patients will do well on this alone.

DO consider knee braces in the knee with very unstable ligaments causing pain on walking.

DON'T assume that the patient's complaint must be due to osteoarthritis because the X-ray confirms the osteoarthritis. Look for other causes such as bursitis, tendinitis, and chronic pain syndromes as well.

DON'T use oral corticosteroids in osteoarthritis.

Section 4 – Localized pain and swelling

Lower part of the algorithm

We will now move into that part of the algorithm in which the answer to the question of objective swelling being present is 'yes'. Remember that the joint swelling must be objectively noted, not just a complaint of the patient's. Some forms of arthritis have episodic swelling, and so it is necessary to have the patient report immediately upon the next episode. Giving a patient a diagnosis of arthritis and starting therapy for such may be doing great harm to someone who does not have arthritis.

Confirming that there is localized pain, and objective evidence for swelling, limits the diagnostic possibilities. They are limited further by noting one or more joints being involved. The following sections start with the patient with monoarthritis, then the patient with polyarthritis, realizing that there are overlaps between the two groups. Thus, crystal arthropathy will be discussed for the two possibilities: monoarticular and polyarticular.

Section 4 – Localized pain and swelling

Palindromic arthritis

If a patient complains of episodic joint pain and swelling lasting a few days, with no symptoms between attacks, they probably have one of three conditions. First, patients with fibromyalgia or other chronic pain syndromes (see the topic on chronic pain syndromes, page 26) often complain of joint swelling, but when examined by a competent physician, no objective swelling is noted. If they do have confirmed swelling, then they either have a crystal arthropathy or palindromic arthritis (discussed below). Crystal arthropathy attacks (e.g. gout) do not resolve completely in less than two days, but palindromic arthritis can, so on the basis of a history of very brief attacks, crystal arthropathy can be ruled out. If the attacks last for more than 2 days, either diagnosis is possible and one needs to examine joint fluid to look for crystals. If the patient gives a clear history of acute arthritis of the first MTP joint with swelling, pain and erythema, then gout can be diagnosed, but in other joints, fluid analysis for crystals is needed.

Algorithmic Approach

The patient complains of well-localized pain, involving one joint at a time. He states he has had swelling too. You do not believe him and insist he return when he has swelling. He does, and he has one swollen wrist.

According to the algorithm you have entered the arthritis zone. With one joint involved he must have one of: palindromic arthritis; crystal arthropathy; or septic arthritis.

You note that his swelling and pain comes and goes completely within 24 hours, so it is not a crystal arthropathy. You note that he has had recurrent attacks, so it is not septic arthritis. The diagnosis is palindromic arthritis. If this was the first attack, and lasted 3 days, you would have to aspirate the joint to look for crystals and rule out septic arthritis.

Palindromic arthritis produces, as the name suggests, attacks that leave the patient the same following the attack as prior to the attack; that is completely well. Symptoms of pain, swelling, erythema, and stiffness may develop over be affected at different times. The time between attacks may be quite variable (days to months). At least 50% of these patients will go on to develop rheumatoid arthritis (after months or years). Rarely they will eventually turn out to develop SLE.

Laboratory measures of inflammation (e.g. ESR) will be normal between attacks, and X-rays will show only soft tissue swelling, and no other changes.

One may use NSAIDs to treat acute attacks, but often the attacks are too short-lived for this to be useful. There may be some benefit in using antimalarials, as they may reduce the risk of progression to rheumatoid arthritis as well as provide prophylaxis for future attacks. Doses of chloroquine 250 mg daily (not available in the United States) or hydroxychloroquine 200–400 mg daily may be tried.

DOs and DON'Ts of Palindromic Arthritis

DO consider this diagnosis in any patient who has recurrent acute swelling that resolves completely in 1–4 days and especially if the attacks last only one day or less.

DO ask the patient to contact you when an attack occurs so that it can be objectively confirmed.

DO aspirate to look for uric acid or calcium pyrophosphate crystals, as gout or pseudogout is in the differential when the attacks last for > 2 days.

DO offer antimalarial therapy when the diagnosis is confirmed.

DON'T assume that the patient is correct when they claim to have joint swelling since patients with chronic pain syndromes often complain of swelling when there is none.

Section 4 – Localized pain and swelling

Crystal arthropathy

When a patient gives a history of an acute attack of joint swelling and marked pain which lasts for a few days, subsides, and is followed by an extended symptom-free interval, consider a crystal arthropathy. The only other possibilities are palindromic arthritis (see the topic on palindromic arthritis, page 100) or a condition where the patient thinks they have swelling, but none is found when they are examined (e.g. fibromyalgia). Whenever a patient claims to have swelling not seen by the physician, an arrangement should be made for the patient to contact a physician when an attack occurs, so that objective swelling can be proven, and fluid aspirated for crystal analysis.

Attacks of proven joint swelling that completely resolve in less than 48 hours do not represent a crystal arthropathy. Rather they more likely represent palindromic arthritis.

Algorithmic Approach

The patient will describe well-localized pain, and complain of swelling. When you document that swelling is present, you have entered the arthritis zone.

According to the algorithm, with only one swollen joint, the patient must have one of: palindromic arthritis; crystal arthropathy; or septic arthritis.

The episode has been present for three days. You read about palindromic arthritis, and decide that this is not the case here. You (or someone) must aspirate the joint to rule out septic arthritis and look for crystals. (It is true that when a man walks in with the first toe swollen and red, he has gout, but any other scenario requires confirmation.)

Had the patient presented with swelling in more than one joint, as crystal arthropathy may, then according to the algorithm they must have one of: rheumatoid arthritis; SLE; spondyloarthropathy; or crystal arthropathy.

The first three are addressed easily by asking questions regarding, and examining for, the diagnostic criteria. (Do not order X-rays for the spondyloarthropathy unless the clinical criteria are evident.) Crystal arthropathy requires aspiration for diagnosis.

Erythema with acute synovitis generally only occurs in crystal arthropathy or septic arthritis.

The crystal arthropathies are a group of diseases in which deposition of crystals and the inflammatory response to these crystals in the joint are chiefly responsible for the arthritis. As stated previously, such crystals may be found in asymptomatic patients, and in osteoarthritic joints. The exact mechanisms by which these crystals are deposited and induce the inflammatory response is not entirely understood. The three most common crystal arthropathies are due to urate crystals (gout), calcium pyrophosphate crystals (pseudogout), and calcium hydroxyapatite crystals. They are an important group to consider in the differential diagnosis of inflammatory arthritis, particularly gout, which may mimic rheumatoid arthritis. The key to their diagnosis is in the demonstration of crystals in synovial fluid, but because such a finding may not always be responsible for disease, it is important to assess whether or not the patient's symptoms are in keeping with a crystal arthropathy, as discussed below.

Gout

Gout is due to sodium urate crystal deposition in joints and soft tissues. Thus, bursitis, tendinitis, cellulitis, nephrolithiasis, and arthritis are all manifestations of the disease. Virtually all patients with gouty arthritis have had a period of asymptomatic hyperuricemia prior to their symptoms, but hyperuricemia alone appears to be insufficient for development of the arthritis since the majority of patients with hyperuricemia never develop gout. More importantly, acute attacks of gout are precipitated in any one of high, normal, or low levels of serum uric acid. It may be a sudden change in the concentration of uric acid which is more important in the acute attack. Therefore, the measurement of serum uric acid levels when encountering a patient suspected of having gout is irrelevant in diagnostic considerations – the uric acid level neither confirming nor ruling out the diagnosis.

Hyperuricemia arises from overproduction or decreased excretion or both. Although there is a long list of such causes, decreased excretion is most commonly the result of: (1) a primary, idiopathic reduction in renal excretion, not well understood; (2) virtually all forms of renal insufficiency or failure; or (3) drugs such as diuretics and low-dose acetylsalicylic acid (ASA). Increased uric acid production is a much less common cause, being most commonly: (1) idiopathic; or due to (2) hematologic malignancies; or (3) alcohol use.

Precipitating factors of an acute gouty attack include drugs that change serum uric acid levels. Levels are acutely elevated by alcohol use, and dehydration (including diuretics). They are acutely decreased by allopurinol, probenecid, or sulfapyrazone. Trauma, major illness, surgery, and infection may also precipitate an attack. Diet is not relevant except in individuals consuming massive amounts of purines.

Acute gouty arthritis occurs most commonly in men, and in most cases the first attack is in the MTP joints (particularly the first MTP). **It is rare to see gout in a woman under 50 years old.** Other sites of involvement include the ankle, midfoot, knee, wrist, elbow, interphalangeal joints, olecranon bursa, and patellar tendon. The attack may also be polyarticular. The attacks are often sudden, producing a swollen, erythematous, exquisitely painful joint. The patient may be systemically ill with fever, malaise, anorexia, and nausea. Attacks usually last for a few days, but may last for weeks. A key diagnostic feature is that they resolve spontaneously and completely (although the next attack may closely follow the first). Pruritus and desquamation over the site is sometimes seen.

In time, the patient may develop chronic tophaceous gout characterized by asymmetric joint swelling, solid deposits of urate (tophi) in joints, and in soft tissues (helix of the ear, olecranon or patellar bursa, ulnar surface of forearm, and Achilles tendon).

Chronic uric acid nephropathy is probably not a true entity, but acute urate nephropathy can be related to acute tubular obstruction (e.g. massive amounts of urate produced following chemotherapy). Hypertension is seen in 10–30% of patients with gout. Both uric acid and calcium oxalate nephrolithiasis occur with increased frequency in patients with gout.

The only truly useful test is synovial fluid analysis. During an acute attack, the synovial fluid will be inflammatory (often containing > 25 000 WBC/mm), and with polarized microscopy the typical needle-shaped, negatively birefringent intra- and extra-cellular crystals may be seen. Absence of the crystals does not rule out the diagnosis, but in the absence of a classic history makes it doubtful. The finding of an intracellular (within WBC) crystal is most specific for an acute attack. Between attacks, one may also find crystals, but since crystals can be found and are not necessarily pathogenic in other forms of arthritis, a previous history consistent with gouty attack is important in interpreting this finding. The diagnosis can also be made by aspirating or biopsying a tophus and demonstrating the urate crystals.

If you are wondering whether or not someone has gout, you SHOULD NOT order a serum uric acid level. A diagnosis of gout cannot be made based on an elevated level of uric acid because the vast majority of individuals with hyperuricemia never get gout. A normal or low level of uric acid does not rule out gout. The only way to be sure of gout is to get a classic history of 1st MTP joint attack in a man or to find crystals. Serum uric acid levels are simply not helpful in confirming or excluding the diagnosis of gout.

Radiographs (particularly of the hands or feet) may show 'punched out' (i.e. with a definite, complete bony margin) subperiosteal cysts near the joint, and with long standing disease, joint destruction and ankylosis may be seen. Tophi are usually radiolucent, although some have calcification. It may be difficult to distinguish between rheumatoid arthritis and gout on the basis of radiographs alone.

The treatment of gout is aimed at alleviating the acute attack, treating tophaceous gout, and providing prophylaxis against future attacks. Consideration should be given to the cause of the patient's hyperuricemia if the history suggests diseases causing uric acid overproduction, for example, exist. Asymptomatic hyperuricemia is in itself not an indication for chronic prophylactic therapy since it may take years before symptoms occur, there are adverse effects from drug therapy, and there is no evidence that renal disease will develop prior to the time when arthritis is manifest. The risk of nephrolithiasis in patients with asymptomatic hyperuricemia is much lower than in patients with gout, so that this is seldom used as an indication for prophylaxis.

Weight loss, control of hypertension, and discouraging heavy alcohol intake may be useful. Special dietary changes are rarely helpful. The acute attack may be treated by five methods:

NSAIDs (often indomethacin is chosen)
Oral colchicine
Intravenous colchicine
Intra-articular corticosteroids
Oral corticosteroids

High dose NSAID is used for 4–10 days (high dose ASA, but not low-dose, can be used). This is effective in most cases. In individuals unable to tolerate, or who have contraindications to NSAIDs, one may use colchicine. Oral colchicine is not used often, but can be given as 1 mg initially, then 0.5 mg every 2 h until the attack subsides, the patient develops dose-limiting nausea or diarrhea, or until 8 mg has been given. Intravenous colchicine is given as 2–3 mg as single bolus, being very careful to avoid interstitial injection which may cause tissue necrosis (have an intravenous line which is running freely and secure). One should avoid giving a total dose of more than 4 mg of IV colchicine. Failure to respond to any of these (i.e. within 48 hours) should prompt one to consider another diagnosis (especially infection) or to consider prednisone (prednisolone) 20–30 mg for 4–7 days if the diagnosis is certain. Avoid any agent that alters uric acid levels suddenly, such as probenecid, allopurinol, or sulfapyrazone since they may precipitate another attack. (See case scenarios for treatment of gout in the patient with renal insufficiency, page 110.)

Do not mix oral and IV colchicine since it is difficult to predict the individual's serum colchicine levels following oral administration, and unpredictable acute toxicity may occur. Equally, if a patient has received IV colchicine, oral colchicine should not be given for at least 1 week, with an even longer delay in the presence of renal insufficiency.

After the acute attack, one may consider prophylaxis if the patient has many recurrent attacks, has tophi or joint destruction, renal disease, or nephrolithiasis. Prophylaxis can be achieved using: allopurinol; probenecid; or sulfinpyrazone.

Allopurinol inhibits uric acid production. Start with 100–300 mg qd if the patient has normal renal function (otherwise 100 mg qd) in order to obtain normal serum uric acid levels. Probenecid 0.5–1.0 mg qd or sulfinpyrazone 100 mg tid may be used as they act as uricosuric agents. They are contraindicated, however, in individuals with nephrolithiasis, renal disease, or urinary uric acid excretion of >7.0 mmol/d.

There is a significant likelihood that a patient started on allopurinol or other prophylactic agents will develop attacks in the first 3 months of therapy, so that the patient should be on colchicine 0.6 mg bid or an NSAID when started on allopurinol (preferably a week before starting the allopurinol). The colchicine or NSAIDs are discontinued after the 3 months, if the attacks are no longer occurring and the serum uric acid level is normal. The patient must be clearly told that they have to be on the colchicine or NSAID for this period even though they are not having attacks, otherwise allopurinol will cause attacks early on.

Some prefer to use lower doses of allopurinol in those with renal failure since this may, over the first few months, reduce the incidence of drug hypersensitivity that is a common cause for discontinuing the drug. Doses of 100 mg qd could be used. Colchicine should be given in lower doses (0.6 mg qd) to patients with renal insufficiency to reduce adverse effects and the long term complication of myopathy and neuropathy.

The treatment of nephrolithiasis (assuming the stones are calcium oxalate or uric acid stones) includes liberal water intake, allopurinol (not uricosuric agents), acetazolamide 250 mg bid-tid, or potassium citrate 30–80 mg qd.

Patients should remain on prophylactic therapy with urate-lowering drugs for at least 2 years, and probably indefinitely, since recurrence is otherwise common. Tophi will eventually resolve in the face of ongoing urate-lowering therapy, but this process may take 2–5 years.

Gout rarely affects the shoulder, so look for another cause of shoulder pain (usually supraspinatus tendinitis).

Pseudogout

Calcium pyrophosphate crystal deposition disease may manifest as pseudogout, a pseudo-rheumatoid arthritis disease, and a pseudo-osteoarthritis disease. The term chondrocalcinosis refers to deposition of such crystals in cartilage. While commonly seen in pseudogout, chondrocalcinosis is also seen in asymptomatic individuals, osteoarthritis, primary hyperparathyroidism, hemochromatosis, gout, hypothyroidism, and joint trauma (including surgery). There is no clear defect of overproduction or underexcretion or metabolism of calcium pyrophosphate that explains pseudogout in a fashion as uric acid metabolism relates to gout.

Pseudogout, of course, mimics gout, but the attacks of pseudogout are more likely to resolve over weeks, and pain tends to develop later in the attack, and persist longer when other manifestations are disappearing. It also tends to affect predominantly the knee (most common), shoulder, wrist, and ankles.

The pseudo-rheumatoid arthritis form is distinguished from true rheumatoid arthritis because the former tends to have flares in a less symmetric pattern. Radiographs in the pseudo-rheumatoid arthritis disease may show chondrocalcinosis, osteophytes, and an absence of erosions or periarticular osteopenia. Otherwise, the joint distribution, and morning stiffness may be quite similar.

The pseudo-osteoarthritis form is distinguished from true osteoarthritis because the former tends to involve ankle, wrist, metacarpophalangeal, and shoulder joints. The pseudo-osteoarthritis is often bilateral, often with a history of acute inflammatory episodes, and a unique, marked bony proliferation of the patellofemoral compartment, not usually seen with typical osteoarthritis.

Attacks of pseudogout may be precipitated by an acute illness, trauma, and surgery. Synovial fluid analysis will be similar to gout, but calcium pyrophosphate crystals may sometimes be seen by polarized microscopy in pseudogout. These crystals are polymorphic, most often rhomboid or rectangular, sometimes needle-shaped, and are positively birefringent. They are smaller than uric acid crystals, and more often intra-cellular. Radiographs may also reveal calcification in bursae, tendons, and ligaments. As well, subperiosteal cysts may be seen, as in gout.

Treatment is very much the same as for gout, except systemic corticosteroids are not needed. There is no prophylaxis available. One should consider appropriate investigations if some of the other diseases associated with chondrocalcinosis (like hypothyroidism, hyperparathyroidism, or hemochromatosis) are suspected, but specific treatment of these diseases may not alter the course of calcium pyrophosphate crystal deposition. For the pseudo-rheumatoid arthritis and pseudo-osteoarthritis forms, NSAIDs are used more often chronically.

Hydroxyapatite deposition disease

Calcium phosphate is normally deposited as hydroxyapatite crystals in bone, but can also be associated with disease when deposited in other tissues. Some of these diseases include calcific periarthritis, calcific tendinitis or bursitis, and arthritis. These crystals are also responsible for the calcinosis seen in various rheumatic diseases. The crystals are too small to be seen on light microscopy.

Their tissue deposition is particularly common in patients with renal failure who have high serum phosphate levels (therefore a tendency towards precipitation of the basic calcium phosphate product). Lowering the phosphate level by chronic dialysis, or calcium carbonate (the latter two being absorbers of phosphate in the gut) is often effective in such patients.

Calcific periarthritis is often an acute periarticular swelling which may be monoarticular or polyarticular, and most commonly involves the shoulder, hip, knee, elbow, wrist, and ankle joints, and rarely the first MTP joint. The attack is associated with the appearance radiographically of periarticular calcification, which often resolves as the attack resolves. The treatment is very much the same as for other crystal arthropathies (NSAIDs, colchicine, or intra-articular corticosteroids), but there is no prophylactic therapy. Some individuals require surgical removal of the calcification if conservative therapy has failed to relieve symptoms.

Calcific tendinitis or bursitis produces an acute inflammatory condition that appears much like any other form of tendinitis or bursitis, but the radiographs will show the calcification of hydroxyapatite deposition. Rotator cuff calcification is a common form and produces symptoms typical of impingement syndrome (painful arc of abduction through 60–120°). The natural history is resorption of the calcification within 2 weeks if there is an acute inflammatory episode, so that the patient is treated initially with NSAIDs, or intra-articular or subacromial (subdeltoid) bursa corticosteroids. The calcification may, however, follow a rotator cuff injury and not be the cause of the injury.

An actual arthritis may occur (most commonly in the shoulder), and may become chronic and destructive. The synovial fluid tends to have fewer than 1000 WBC/mm. Radiographs of the shoulder may show glenohumeral joint destruction and significant rotator cuff atrophy (this helps distinguish this condition from simple osteoarthritis of the glenohumeral joint). Treatment is with NSAIDs or analgesics, intra-articular corticosteroids being largely ineffective and possibly detrimental.

Case scenarios of gout

Because the treatment of gout can involve a number of medications, each with their specific uses depending on the pattern of the patient's gout, it is worthwhile to review some scenarios.

First, renal function must always be known when considering therapy with NSAIDs and colchicine. Prednisone (prednisolone) is a last resort and should probably only be used by a rheumatologist in this setting. Use the lower doses of allopurinol and colchicine in patients with renal insufficiency.

When treating gout the diagnosis should be confirmed by crystal identification, and septic arthritis should either be very unlikely or ruled out by culture. If in doubt, since there have been cases of crystals and infection both being present, one can either wait, or treat with non-corticosteroid methods until culture results are known. The therapeutic choices are listed in descending order of choice, but which therapy is used depends on contra-indications also.

Having multiple attacks does not mean prophylaxis is necessary. If the patient is happy to treat each attack as it occurs, then let them be.

1. *A 45-year-old man develops acute, painful, swollen big toe.* The diagnosis of gout is virtually always correct in a man presenting with this complaint, but is not in a woman, where septic arthritis has to be ruled out by aspiration. In other joints, the diagnosis should be confirmed by aspiration. Treat with one of:
   (a) Intra-articular corticosteroid injection;
   (b) NSAID in full dose (e.g. indomethacin 50 mg po tid, tenoxicam 20 mg po qd, diclofenac 50 mg po tid);
   (c) Colchicine 2–3 mg IV × 1, with no further colchicine of any type for at least 1 week (longer delay in those with compromised renal function);
   (d) Colchicine 0.6 mg po q2h until the symptoms are reduced significantly, the total dose of 8 mg orally is reached, or drug is not tolerated (nausea and diarrhea occurs), with no further colchicine of any type for at least 1 week (longer delay in those with compromised renal function);
   (e) Prednisone (prednisolone) 30 mg po qd × 1 week, or prednisolone 80–120 mg IM once.

2. *A 45-year-old man develops an attack of gout while on an NSAID.* First, is the patient on the maximum recommended dose of NSAID? If not, increase their dose. Otherwise treat with one of:
   (a) Intra-articular corticosteroid injection;
   (b) Colchicine 2–3 mg IV × 1, with no further colchicine of any type for at least 1 week (longer delay in those with compromised renal function);
   (c) Colchicine 0.6 mg po q2h until the symptoms are reduced significantly, the total dose of 8 mg orally is reached, or drug is not tolerated (nausea and diarrhea occurs), with no further colchicine of any type for at least 1 week (longer delay in those with compromised renal function);
   (d) Prednisone (prednisolone) 30 mg po qd × 1 week.

3. *A 45-year-old man has been having recurrent attacks for which he takes an NSAID, but he would prefer to have fewer attacks altogether.* If the patient is currently asymptomatic, start prophylaxis with:
   (a) NSAID in moderate dose and allopurinol 100–300 mg po qd (starting the allopurinol after about 1 week of NSAID use);
   (b) Colchicine 0.6 mg po qd-bid and allopurinol 100–300 mg po qd (starting the allopurinol after about 1 week of colchicine use);
   (c) The allopurinol is given in conjunction with the other agent for at least 3 months, after which the NSAID or colchicine can be discontinued

completely, waiting for the possibility of a recurrence in which case it should be restarted.

4. *A 45-year-old man with an attack that resolved 3 days ago and frequent attacks as far as the patient is concerned.* It is acceptable to start allopurinol this soon after an attack only if there will be another agent used in the first week before allopurinol is started and this agent is continued in conjunction with allopurinol for at least 3 months. Treat with one of:
    (a) NSAID in moderate dose and allopurinol 100–300 mg po qd (starting the allopurinol after about 1 week of NSAID use);
    (b) Colchicine 0.6 mg po qd-bid and allopurinol 100–300 mg po qd (starting the allopurinol after about 1 week of colchicine use).

5. *A 45-year-old man has an attack of gout despite the fact that he has been on allopurinol (now on its own).* Treat with one of:
    (a) Intra-articular corticosteroid injection;
    (b) NSAID in full dose (e.g. indomethacin 50 mg po tid, tenoxicam 20 mg po qd, diclofenac 50 mg po tid) for about 1 week;
    (c) Colchicine 2–3 mg IV × 1, with no further colchicine of any type for at least 1 week (longer delay in those with compromised renal function);
    (d) Colchicine 0.6 mg po q2h until the symptoms are reduced significantly, the total dose of 8 mg orally is reached, or drug is not tolerated (nausea and diarrhea occurs), with no further colchicine of any type for at least 1 week (longer delay in those with compromised renal function);
    (e) Prednisone (prednisolone) 30 mg po qd × 1 week.

6. *A 45-year-old man has ongoing attacks or persistent attacks when on allopurinol, and despite attempts to treat each attack.* STOP the allopurinol, and start one of:
    (a) Intra-articular corticosteroid injection if not yet tried;
    (b) NSAID in full dose if not yet tried;
    (c) Colchicine 2–3 mg IV × 1, with no further colchicine of any type for at least 1 week (longer delay in those with compromised renal function), if no recent use of colchicine;
    (d) Colchicine 0.6 mg po q2h until the symptoms are reduced significantly, the total dose of 8 mg orally is reached, or drug is not tolerated (nausea and diarrhea occurs), if no recent use of colchicine. No further colchicine of any type for at least 1 week (longer delay in those with compromised renal function;
    (e) Prednisone (prednisolone) 30 mg po qd × 2 weeks.

7. *A patient with renal insufficiency develops gout.* Avoid NSAIDs, and do not give more than 1 mg of IV colchicine to anyone with a creatinine over 180 μmol/l (2 mg/dl).

The best option is corticosteroid injection into the joints. If a joint cannot easily be injected into (e.g. forefoot), then systemic corticosteroids such as prednisone (prednisolone) 30 mg po qd for a week, prednisolone 80–120 mg IM once, or methylprednisolone 125 mg IV once, can be tried.

It may also be worthwhile to have a rheumatologist involved if such management is difficult.

Realize that for future prophylaxis, probenecid and sulfinpyrazone are ineffective in renal insufficiency, and that allopurinol should be given at a low dosage (100 mg qd).

DOs and DON'Ts of Crystal Arthropathy

DO aspirate any symptomatic joint with acute or chronic arthritis and look for urate (gout) or calcium pyrophosphate (pseudogout) to confirm the suspected diagnosis.

DO have the patient contact you when they have acute joint swelling so that it can be confirmed objectively.

DO consider palindromic arthritis in the differential diagnosis of crystal arthropathy (and suspect it when attacks completely resolve in less than 2 days).

DO order X-rays of the joint suspected of having crystal arthropathy and look for chondrocalcinosis (seen in pseudogout).

DO discontinue or lower dose of diuretics in the patient if possible.

DO consider allopurinol prophylaxis in the patient with tophi (subcutaneous yellow-white lumps or uric acid crystals), or with too many or too prolonged attacks for the patient's liking.

DO put the patient on some anti-inflammatory agent (an NSAID or colchicine 0.6 mg bid) on a regular basis, before starting allopurinol prophylaxis. Maintain the anti-inflammatory agent for at least 3–6 months before allowing the patient to remain on allopurinol alone. Otherwise allopurinol will induce acute attacks during this period.

DO prescribe lower doses of allopurinol or colchicine in patients with renal insufficiency.

DON'T measure serum uric acid to try to determine whether or not a patient has gout; it is not useful. A normal or low uric acid does not rule out gout and a high uric acid does not mean gout.

DON'T treat asymptomatic hyperuricemia (many patients on diuretics will have hyperuricemia).

DON'T diagnose gout unless one has a classic history of acute attacks (days) of 1st MTP joint or dorsal foot synovitis (sudden onset, severe, erythema, swelling, desquamation, resolving in a few days) or uric acid crystals have been found.

DON'T diagnose pseudogout in the absence of crystals identified in synovial fluid or chondrocalcinosis on X-ray.

DON'T clinically diagnose gout in a women under 40 years old (even if it affects the 1st MTP joint) since such events are truly rare in young women, and infection is more likely the cause in their case.

DON'T start allopurinol without an anti-inflammatory agent for the first 3–6 months at least, or acute attacks will be precipitated.

DON'T mix oral and intravenous colchicine.

DON'T attribute shoulder pain to gout.

Section 4 – Localized pain and swelling

Septic arthritis

Whenever a patient presents with monoarthritis, septic arthritis must be considered. To miss septic arthritis is to cause probable joint destruction. Erythema is an important sign in arthritis. When erythema is present, it can only mean one of three things: cellulitis; septic arthritis; or crystal arthropathy. With cellulitis, the range of motion of the joint is near normal, because the joint is not involved. With septic arthritis the range of motion of the joint will never be entirely normal. In fact, when the joint cannot be moved at all, this is septic arthritis until proven otherwise.

Algorithmic Approach

The patient will complain of well localized pain. It will be relatively easy to detect swelling. Septic arthritis is almost always one joint, but occasional cases involving more than one joint do occur. In such cases, the patient is quite ill, and in severe pain.

The algorithm brings you to the arthritis zone, and with one joint involved, the patient must have one of: palindromic arthritis; crystal arthropathy; or septic arthritis.

Joint aspiration is necessary for the latter two, and only if these are ruled out is one prepared to make the diagnosis of palindromic arthritis when the patient is in the middle of their first episode. (An episode that has come and gone is not septic arthritis.)

The only way to separate crystal arthritis from septic arthritis is either if pain, swelling, and erythema are clearly resolving without any sort of therapy, or by joint fluid analysis. No one will ever be critical of the physician who aspirates (or arranges for someone else to aspirate) joint fluid and submit it for Gram stain, culture, and crystal analysis. When one thinks the chance of septic arthritis is low (e.g. pain and swelling for more than 2 weeks, near normal range of motion) one could wait 24 h for culture results and observe the patient as an outpatient. If not as sure, however, the patient should be observed in hospital while awaiting culture results. It is also acceptable to obtain joint fluid, and begin IV antibiotics in hospital. One can stop the antibiotics after cultures are negative for 48 h and observe the patient further off antibiotics.

If one has difficulty with obtaining joint fluid initially, refer to someone who can. If arthrocentesis still proves difficult, the options are to observe the patient in hospital for another day (as crystal arthropathies normally show some improvement). An NSAID can be given during this in-hospital observation, which may make a very significant difference in crystal arthritis, but will not significantly affect septic arthritis. Corticosteroid injection is not recommended, since it may significantly improve the symptoms of septic arthritis only to have joint destruction continue, and symptoms recur in a few days. An alternative to in-hospital observation for 24–48 h, is to have a surgeon perform an arthrotomy or arthroscopy to rule out septic arthritis, but obviously this is less preferable.

With this general approach, septic arthritis will rarely be missed. Obtaining a WBC count cannot substitute for obtaining joint fluid. A normal WBC count does not rule out septic arthritis, especially in the elderly. An elevated WBC count can be seen in both crystal arthropathy and septic arthritis. Absence of fever in no way rules out septic arthritis. Remember that one is never allowed to miss septic arthritis, so obtain joint fluid, or at least either observe the patient in hospital, or get a second opinion.

As to the treatment of bacterial septic arthritis, IV antibiotics are necessary. There is debate and some differences among physicians on how long to use IV antibiotics. Some recommend at least 4–6 weeks IV and possibly 2 weeks oral therapy to follow. Others suggest only 2 weeks IV and 2–4 weeks oral. **All forms of septic arthritis must be drained**. The knee joint can sometimes be drained by repeated arthrocentesis (every 1–2 days) until there is no effusion, and the patient remains asymptomatic on antibiotics. Other joints, however, cannot easily be drained by aspiration, and require surgical drainage.

The choice of antibiotic in most cases is empirically one that covers *Staphylococcus aureus*, and streptococcal species. Flucloxacillin (1.0–2.0 g IV q6h in an adult) or cefazolin (1.5–2.0 g IV q8h in an adult with normal renal function) are acceptable choices, until culture results and sensitivities are obtained (Cefuroxime 1.5 g IV q8h is used in the UK instead of cefazolin.). In patients known to have a prosthesis or access for *Staphylococcal epidermidis* (like a central line or a patient on hemodialysis), vancomycin is recommended instead, until culture results are known. Antibiotics should be started after joint fluid is obtained, otherwise a false-negative culture may occur (normally > 95% of bacterial septic arthritis is culture-positive). The Gram stain helps to choose antibiotics initially. In immunosuppressed patients (e.g. patients with neutropenia, hematologic malignancy, AIDS) and intravenous drug abusers, Gram-negative coverage is used empirically (either ceftazidime or an aminoglycoside and pipercillin).

Gonococcal arthritis is the most common form of septic arthritis in young adults who are sexually active, and therefore must be the first consideration in this age group. Since it is very uncommon to obtain a positive culture from joint fluid in this form of septic arthritis, one has to sometimes treat monoarthritis in this age group empirically with antibiotics after joint aspiration to rule out other organisms as a potential cause. The source of infection may be urethritis, cervicitis, pharyngitis, and proctitis, so these areas should be swabbed, depending on the individual's sexual practices, even if there are no symptoms from that body region. Reiter's syndrome can be distinguished from this form of septic arthritis by the presence of gradual onset (several days) back pain, conjunctivitis, painless oral ulcers, diarrhea, and psoriasiform rash on palm and soles in Reiter's syndrome. Treat with a few days to a week of IV penicillin 3 million units q4h or ceftriaxone 1.0 g IV or IM q24h, then oral penicillin to complete 2 weeks of therapy.

Septic bursitis is approached similarly to septic arthritis, although antibiotic therapy for a total of 2 weeks is usually sufficient (perhaps 4 weeks for olecranon bursitis).

As soon as the patient's pain is improved, and the joint drained, begin mobilizing the joint to prevent contractures.

In a patient with a persistent monoarthritis for weeks to months, with no evidence of bacterial infection or crystal arthropathy on fluid analysis, one should consider tuberculous (TB) infection if they have the risk factors (known to have TB previously, a member of TB-endemic population). The diagnosis normally requires surgical synovial biopsy and culturing for mycobacteria. As well, Lyme disease should be considered in patients with persistent monoarthritis who live, or have been in, endemic areas: in Canada (Lake Erie); in the United States (Northeast and West coast, and the upper Midwest); or in Central Europe.

Prosthetic joint infections should be managed with input from an orthopedic surgeon, and infectious diseases consultant. The key diagnostic problem with prosthetic joints is that septic arthritis may not be as clinically apparent in these joints, and often it is difficult to be sure whether or not pain in the joint is related to loosening of the prosthesis or to infection. One approach to this diagnostic problem is to perform a bone scan. If the bone scan is negative, and the patient has not received therapy, infection is not a concern. If the bone scan is positive, one should perform a gallium (or other inflammatory) scan to rule out infection. The patient must not be on antibiotics, since a false-negative scan may be obtained in this setting. In some cases, it is possible to suppress the infection with antibiotics chronically and allow the patient to retain the prosthesis rather than undertake surgical removal, a consideration to be discussed with a surgeon.

DOs and DON'Ts of Septic Arthritis

DO suspect this in any acute (< 1 week) monoarthritis, especially when there is erythema and marked restriction of motion, and try to obtain synovial fluid. Consult a rheumatologist or orthopedic surgeon if fluid cannot be obtained.

DO rule out tuberculous infection when an unexplained monoarthritis persists in a patient at risk for such infections (someone from a TB-endemic area, within known history of a TB, or with immunodeficiency).

DON'T accept gout as the diagnosis in a woman (even if the 1st MTP joint is involved), unless she is over 40 and has some good reason for developing it (e.g. renal disease, diuretics). Look for septic arthritis.

DON'T accept acute monoarthritis in a patient with a systemic arthritis (like rheumatoid arthritis or SLE) as being just some sort of flare. Look for infection when only one joint is involved.

DON'T treat septic arthritis with oral antibiotics from the start.

DON'T fail to aspirate a joint suspected of having infection and merely commit the patient to an entire course (which might be up to 6 weeks) of antibiotics, not knowing what disease the patient actually has.

Section 4 – Localized pain and swelling

Rheumatoid arthritis

Rheumatoid arthritis is a chronic, systemic inflammatory disease of unknown etiology, characterized by typical symmetric arthritis of the hands and feet, particularly the PIP and MCP joints, with bone erosion.

Algorithmic Approach

The patient has complained of pain that is localized, so you are now traveling down the algorithm. The patient complains of swelling and you notice that there actually is swelling. The patient has more than one joint involved and so according to the algorithm you know they must have one of: rheumatoid arthritis; SLE; spondyloarthropathy; or crystal arthropathy.

Now go to the diagnostic criteria for the first three to obtain the questions on history and the findings on examination that should be sought for each.

Morning stiffness > 1 ?	Yes
Arthritis of at least three joints?	Yes
Arthritis of the hand joints?	Yes
Symmetric arthritis?	Yes
Rheumatoid nodule	No
Rheumatoid factor	Negative
Joint erosions on X-ray?	No

(Symptoms must be present for more than 6 weeks.)

Diagnosis made: rheumatoid arthritis. To rule out SLE:

Malar, discoid or photosensitive rash?	No
Oral ulcers?	No
Arthritis of more than two joints	Yes

Serositis (pleuritis, pericarditis)	No
Renal disease (laboratory)	No
Hematologic disorder (laboratory)	No
Serology	Serology for SLE is not required when the patient has only one criterion

And if you want to rule out a spondyloarthropathy:

Nocturnal pain or morning stiffness of lumbar or dorsal spine?	No
Asymmetric arthritis?	No
Alternating right and left buttock pain?	No
Sausage digit?	No
Plantar fasciitis?	Yes
Iritis or conjunctivitis?	No
Urethritis?	No
Any of psoriasis, balanitis, or inflammatory bowel disease?	No
Positive family history?	No
HLA-B27 positive? (Do not order X-rays for the spondyloarthropathy unless the clinical criteria are evident.)	This test is not required

Finally, you may aspirate a joint to look for crystals. In any case, the algorithmic approach brought you to four possibilities in this patient complaining of joint pain with swelling. These are easily separated by diagnostic criteria and aspiration.

Clinical manifestations

Constitutional symptoms including fatigue, fever, weight loss, weakness, and myalgias are often seen. In fact, weight loss of as much as 10 kg can occur when the disease is very active. The disease usually appears insidiously, but the clinical course is highly variable. In the majority of patients, however, remission is rare and progressive joint erosions and deformity occurs. Morning stiffness of more than one hour is almost invariably seen in inflammatory arthritis, and may be even more prolonged in rheumatoid arthritis.

Joint swelling may be quite pronounced, and the arthritis may affect many synovial joints including sternoclavicular, acromioclavicular, and temporo-mandibular joints. The cervical spine may be involved. A number of extra-articular manifestations also occur as listed in *Table 4.1* below.

Deformities include radial deviation at the wrist, ulnar deviation at MCP joints, palmar subluxation of proximal phalanges, swan-neck deformity (hyperexten-sion of PIP with flexion of DIP), boutonnière deformity (flexion of PIP, extension of DIP), hyperextension of first IP joint with flexion of first MCP (causing loss of thumb mobility and pinch), metatarsal prolapse, arch collapse, hallux valgus, and atlantoaxial subluxation.

Tenosynovitis and bursitis commonly accompany the joint disease. Examples include rotator cuff tendinitis, subacromial (subdeltoid) bursitis, elbow epicondylitis ('tennis' and 'golfer's' elbow), De Quervain's tenosynovitis (abductor pollicus longus and extensor pollicus brevis), hand extensor and flexor tenosynovitis, and trochanteric bursitis of the lower limb. Extensor tenosyn-ovitis of the hands is an important complication since chronic involvement (> 6 months), disuse atrophy, and mechanical trauma on the ulnar styloid predis-pose to spontaneous tendon rupture, leading to further dysfunction of an already functionally impaired hand. Prophylactic surgery may be useful when the tendinitis has become chronic (> 3 months) and is not responding to medical therapy.

Cervical spine involvement generally occurs in those who have erosions in the hands and feet. The laxity of the cruciate ligament supporting the atlantoaxial joint of the cervical spine, together with synovitis of the facet joints is partic-ularly important because it may lead to cervical myelopathy, and if atlantoaxial dissociation is significant, even sudden death. This subluxation is identified by lateral flexion and extension cervical X-rays demonstrating an increase in the distance between the posterior aspect of the C1 vertebral body and the ante-rior aspect of the odontoid process of C2. Normally it should not exceed 3 mm in flexion. The decision as to when spine fusion is indicated to prevent or retard cervical myelopathy is a difficult one since many patients will have subluxation of > 10 mm with no symptoms, and the surgery is difficult and potentially dangerous.

Worrying symptoms (and reasonable indications for surgery) include severe neck pain, numbness in hands or feet, progressive motor symptoms, and urinary retention or incontinence. Most patients have pain rather than neurologic symp-toms. If this pain fails to respond to primary treatment of the disease and immobilization, some patients are candidates for surgery on this basis alone. In addition, it is inadvisable to prescribe neck traction for cervical pain in patients with rheumatoid arthritis and X-ray evidence of C1–C2 subluxation. Active range of motion exercises are considered safe. It is important for an anesthetist to be aware that a patient has rheumatoid arthritis so that for any

Table 4.1 The extra-articular manifestations of rheumatoid arthritis

Skin
>   Palmar erythema
>   Subcutaneous nodules
>   Vasculitis

Lung
>   Pleurisy, pleural effusions
>   Pneumonitis
>   Lung nodules
>   Bronchiolitis obliterans

Heart
>   Pericarditis, pericardial effusions
>   Valvular disease
>   Myocarditis

Neuromuscular
>   Nerve entrapment
>   Cervical cord compression
>   Muscle wasting
>   Mononeuritis multiplex
>   Diffuse peripheral neuropathy

Ocular
>   Episcleritis
>   Scleritis, scleromalacia perforans
>   Melting cornea syndrome

Hematologic
>   Normocytic, normochromic anemia
>   Felty's syndrome
>   Amyloidosis

Miscellaneous
>   Sjögren's syndrome
>   Pulmonary infections, septic arthritis
>   Osteoporosis
>   Tenosynovitis
>   Bursitis

Drug-related
>   (see section on drug therapy, page 193)

surgery, appropriate protective measures regarding neck manipulation can be taken during intubation.

Rheumatoid nodules are seen in 20% of patients at some time, usually on the extensor surfaces of the limbs, and particularly at sites chronically exposed to pressure, but may also occur in visceral organs. They are usually not painful, but can be in the pressure areas of the skin surface. With repeated trauma, they may ulcerate and be a portal of infection, or more sinister, their spontaneous ulceration may herald a necrotizing vasculitis. The nodules may involve tendons and nerves, and the sclera (scleromalacia perforans). Their removal for cosmetic reasons is not often recommended since they tend to recur. Similarly, one may try intra-lesional corticosteroid, but again recurrence is common.

Vasculitis is uncommon in rheumatoid arthritis, and generally occurs in patients who have suffered many years with severe disease. It manifests as mononeuritis multiplex, peripheral gangrene, subcutaneous nodule ulceration, renal vasculitis, or even as unexplained weight loss. It is associated with high mortality, so aggressive therapy (corticosteroids and possibly cyclophosphamide) is prescribed when a diagnosis (by biopsy) is made.

Pleural effusions may or may not be accompanied by pleuritis, and can be quite large. They are characteristically associated with (compared with serum) a low glucose level, high lactate dehydrogenase level, and high cholesterol level. These patients should receive full investigation for malignancy or infection as a potential cause, however, before the effusion is ascribed to rheumatoid arthritis. While interstitial pneumonitis may be a manifestation of the disease, in its acute form with fever and cough it is usually a complication of gold and methotrexate therapy, whereas the chronic insidious form is usually due to the disease itself. Similarly, bronchiolitis obliterans may be related to the disease, but has also been associated with gold, penicillamine, and sulfasalazine. It is difficult to separate out the cause of these pulmonary complications, so one is often obligated to withdraw the potentially offending drug. For the interstitial pneumonitis due to rheumatoid arthritis or drugs, treatment with prednisone (prednisolene) is often used. For bronchiolitis obliterans, in which the course is often rapid and fatal, no effective therapy is available, although corticosteroids and cyclophosphamide are tried.

Pericardial effusions are similar pathologically to pleural effusions, and may be associated with pericarditis. Uncomplicated pericarditis (not constrictive) usually responds to corticosteroid treatment alone. Myocarditis is rare, and valvular disease is usually not clinically significant.

Nerve involvement includes carpal tunnel syndrome, ulnar nerve entrapment at wrist or elbow, and the rare mononeuritis multiplex in the setting of vasculitis. The central nervous system is rarely involved, except in cervical compression myelopathy.

Episcleritis manifests as an uncomfortable, sometimes painful, eye condition with red-purple circular lesions near the corneal limbus, surrounded by conjunctival hyperemia. It is treated with topical corticosteroids. Scleritis is rarer and is differentiated from episcleritis by the presence of nodules in the former. It is very painful, associated with systemic vasculitis, and carries with it the risk of orbital rupture. If in doubt, one should refer to an ophthalmologist when eye manifestations appear.

Lymphadenopathy is well described, but tends to correlate with disease activity. Marked adenopathy, particularly without significant evidence for active synovitis, warrants further investigation for neoplasia. Felty's syndrome is the association of neutropenia, anemia, and splenomegaly. It may produce marked neutropenia and an anemia that is more severe than usually seen in rheumatoid arthritis. The spleen is not always palpable however. Platelet count is usually normal or slightly reduced. The bone marrow may be hypocellular, normocellular, or hypercellular. When patients develop Felty's syndrome, they often have an abatement of their arthritis, and can sometimes have drug therapy withdrawn. They are at risk for vasculitis (neuropathy, leg ulcers, scleritis) and for staphylococcal infections (although the latter is not as frequent as one might expect for the degree of neutropenia). Treatment regimens have included gold therapy, or cyclophosphamide with prednisone (prednisolone) if the patient has recurrent infections or vasculitis. Patients who are asymptomatic may be simply followed.

Rheumatoid arthritis does appear to predispose the patient to infections, predominantly pulmonary, so that fever in a patient in the absence of active synovitis, and particularly if high fever, should be assumed to be related to infection. Septic arthritis should be suspected in the patient who presents with significant flare in one joint only.

Patients with rheumatoid arthritis are at greater risk than the general population for hematologic malignancies. Malignancy should be considered if the patient develops unexplained adenopathy or constitutional symptoms when the disease is not very active.

Laboratory findings

Anemia of chronic disease is, of course, common and related to disease activity, often improving with therapy. Thrombocytosis is also seen with active disease. Acute phase reactants (e.g. erythrocyte sedimentation rate, C-reactive protein) are often elevated. Rheumatoid factor may be negative early in the disease, appearing months to years later or not at all. Titers often diminish with therapy.

The important radiographic findings are bone erosions near the articular margins, as their presence contributes to diagnosis. The erosive changes may be asymptomatic, and not necessarily correlated with the activity or degree of synovitis. They are not entirely specific for rheumatoid arthritis as they may occur in the seronegative spondyloarthropathies. They must also be distinguished from the subperiosteal cysts of gout. It is not strictly necessary to obtain a series of radiographs whenever a patient has a major flare, or when a change in therapy is planned. Some argue that one should survey periodically for bone erosions, since their appearance would give reason to change slow-acting anti-rheumatic drugs.

Other than prior to surgery with general anesthesia is not clear whether or not one should periodically obtain cervical spine films, particularly in the asymptomatic patient, unless one is going to include degree of atlantoaxial subluxation as a consideration in determining the need for spine fusion.

Treatment

Begin with education on the need for chronic therapy, and the importance of compliance.

Drug therapy with NSAIDs, corticosteroids, and the slow-acting anti-rheumatic drugs (some object to the term remittive or disease-modifying drugs, since remission in rheumatoid arthritis is quite unusual, and disease modification has not been clearly proven) is discussed in detail later, as it pertains to many rheumatic diseases.

In brief, start slow-acting anti-rheumatic drugs early (when the diagnosis is proven), and use NSAIDs and/or corticosteroid joint injections as a measure to control the disease while waiting for a complete response to the long-term agents. Some assessment of disease activity by counting the number of swollen and tender joints, the degree of morning stiffness, and the overall function and sense of well-being of the patient should be documented. This allows one objectively to judge the patient's response to therapy at a later date, and to decide if a change in therapy is needed.

If it is not entirely clear which form of arthritis the patient has, it is reasonable to treat with NSAIDs initially, but once the diagnosis of rheumatoid arthritis is confirmed (i.e. meets ACR criteria), slow-acting anti-rheumatic drug therapy is recommended.

Use a physiotherapist to instruct on exercises that maintain range of motion and stretching, and an occupational therapist to provide suggestions on how the patient can modify their activity and surroundings to maintain optimum function. As well, splints help to redistribute forces over more than one joint, and gadgets can be helpful when hand function is limited by pain or deformity. Cervical collars may be helpful for patients with cervical pain, although patients must wear them at night only. Constant use leads to atrophy of the neck muscles, and the need for further neck support, only serving to worsen the situation. Periodic collar use and neck strengthening exercises are more effective in the long term.

Look for bunions or bunionettes (which can be treated with wide shoes), provide foot orthoses such as metatarsal pads or custom designed insoles (arch supports) for arch collapse, and a deep toe box for claw toes.

Surgical intervention comes in the form of joint replacements, dorsal wrist tenosynovectomy, carpal tunnel releases, joint fusion, and correction of foot deformities. Correction of hand deformities in rheumatoid patients is often not successful, since current surgical methods rely on soft tissues to stabilize the joint position, and deformities tend to recur.

DOs and DON'Ts of Rheumatoid Arthritis

DO start the patient who has definite rheumatoid arthritis (e.g. if they meet ACR criteria) on a slow-acting anti-rheumatic drug, rather than only treating with NSAIDs alone.

DO examine the feet at each visit and recommend wide shoes and arch supports before deformities become marked.

DO have a plan for restarting a slow-acting anti-rheumatic drug or changing drugs if a problem develops with one drug.

DON'T routinely use oral corticosteroids.

DON'T assume that pain in a patient with rheumatoid arthritis is always due to a flare of arthritis. Look for evidence of tendinitis, bursitis, carpal tunnel syndrome, and chronic pain syndromes as possible considerations. Flares in rheumatoid arthritis almost always produce joint swelling.

Section 4 – Localized pain and swelling

Systemic lupus erythematosus (SLE)

SLE is an inflammatory disease of unknown etiology in which tissues are damaged (possibly) by deposition of pathogenic autoantibodies and immune complexes. Women are more often affected than men, and usually around the age of 20–30 years, but both children and elderly can be affected.

Algorithmic Approach

Scenario 1. A patient with SLE presents without joint swelling. The patient has complained of pain in her hands and feet, and you have insisted that she describe its location exactly. You are convinced that the pain is well localized, so you are now traveling down the algorithm. **Stop! Are you sure you spent enough time asking about the location of the pain? Do not make the mistake of diagnosing a patient with fibromyalgia as having SLE.**

The patient does not complain of swelling and you notice that there actually is no swelling. If you are sure you belong on the left side of the algorithm, then according to the algorithm you know she must have one of: tendinitis/bursitis; osteoarthritis; or SLE.

Now proceed to the diagnostic criteria of SLE, and review the topics on the painful hand and the painful foot or ankle, and osteoarthritis on pages 83, and 92, respectively. The diagnostic criteria will tell you if she has SLE.

Malar, discoid or photosensitive rash?	Yes
Oral ulcers?	No
Arthritis of more than two joints	Yes
Serositis (pleuritis, pericarditis)	No
CNS disorder?	No
Renal disease (laboratory)	Yes
Hematologic disorder (laboratory)	No
Serology	ANA +

Four criteria to confirm diagnosis.

Clinical manifestations and treatment

Systemic symptoms include fatigue, weight loss, and fever. See *Table 4.2* for a list of the manifestations discussed below.

The 'butterfly' rash is a flat or slightly raised, erythematous rash over the cheeks that spares the nasolabial folds (a useful feature in distinguishing it from seborrheic dermatitis) and is the most common dermatologic manifestation. Another common rash is a nonspecific maculopapular rash related to sun exposure, and typically occurring over chest and face (but may occur anywhere). The lesions resolve spontaneously in most cases, but may persist, enlarge, with central atrophy and thus evolve into the lesion of subacute cutaneous lupus. Patients tend to also have photosensitive rash on sun-exposed areas only, and sun exposure may not only lead to the rash, but may precipitate systemic flares. None of these rashes result in scarring, unlike discoid lupus which is an erythematous papule or plaque on the head and neck that leaves central atrophy, scarring, and hyperpigmentation. Skin vasculitis may manifest as ulcers, purpuric lesions (leukocytoclastic vasculitis), splinter hemorrhages, urticaria, and livedo reticularis. They tend to occur in the presence of active disease elsewhere. Oral ulcers are an important diagnostic criterion, but must be looked for closely, as they are often painless.

The malar rash, photosensitivity, and discoid rash respond well to anti-malarials (hydroxychloroquine 400 mg qd or chloroquine 250 mg qd, the latter not available in the United States) or to low dose prednisone (prednisolone) (< 20 mg). The former is preferred so as to avoid chronic corticosteroid use if possible, but corticosteroids may be necessary while awaiting the benefit of

Table 4.2 The clinical manifestations of systemic lupus erythematosus (SLE)

Skin
- Malar rash[a]
- Photosensitivity[a]
- Maculopapular truncal rash
- Discoid lesion[a]
- Splinter hemorrhages
- Alopecia

Musculoskeletal
- Non-erosive arthritis[a]
- Arthralgias
- Myalgias
- Calcinosis
- Avascular necrosis (corticosteroid related)

Cardiovascular
- Postpartum flare
- Raynaud's phenomenon
- Pericarditis[a]
- Myocarditis
- Marantic (Libman-Sacks) endocarditis

Pulmonary
- Pleuritis[a]
- Pleural effusions
- Interstitial fibrosis
- Pneumonitis
- Pulmonary hypertension

Neurologic
- Peripheral neuropathy
- Cranial neuropathy
- Psychosis[a]
- Seizures[a]

Ocular
- Episcleritis
- Conjunctivitis

Hematologic
- Anemia of chronic disease
- Coomb's-positive hemolytic anemia[a]
- Leukopenia or lymphopenia[a]
- Thrombocytopenia[a]
- Splenomegaly
- Prolonged partial thromboplastic time
- Clotting factor inhibitors

Gynecologic
- Spontaneous abortion/still birth
- Amenorrhea
- Postpartum flare
- Neonatal SLE

Miscellaneous
- Anti-phospholipid syndrome
- Lymphadenopathy

[a] Diagnostic criteria.

anti-malarials which may take several weeks. After several months, the dose of hydroxychloroquine could be reduced to 200 mg qd (or chloroquine to alternate day), but it is probably best to continue the drug indefinitely, since patients tend to have flares when it is discontinued. Photosensitivity is also treated by avoiding sunlight overexposure, and using sunscreens (factor strength $\geq$ 15).

The arthritis is almost always nonerosive, but may produce ulnar deviation and morning stiffness, thus mimicking rheumatoid arthritis. The arthritis (as well as arthralgias or myalgias) responds well to NSAIDs or anti-malarials. In some cases, low dose prednisone (prednisolone) may be needed. If the patient develops acute pain in a single joint however, one should consider septic arthritis, or avascular necrosis as causes.

Patients may develop an acute pneumonitis characterized by fever, cough, and dyspnea. This is a diagnosis of exclusion, however, and the presence of pulmonary infiltrates or effusions warrant investigation for an infectious etiology, before concluding it is due to SLE itself. The treatment for pneumonitis or pleuritis is prednisone (prednisolone) 40 mg qd tapered over several weeks to months. Pericarditis and peritonitis due to SLE are also diagnoses of exclusion and are treated as for pleuritis. Pulmonary hypertension may be due to a variety of causes including pulmonary vascular disease, multiple pulmonary emboli, and primary lupus cardiac disease. It may be difficult to treat, but cyclophosphamide, and high-dose corticosteroids have been used.

The renal disease of SLE includes minimal change disease, membranous glomerulonephritis, membranoproliferative glomerulonephritis, diffuse proliferative glomerulonephritis (the most serious), and mesangial proliferative glomerulonephritis. Patients should have a urinalysis at the time of diagnosis, and then at regular intervals (e.g. 6 months). If proteinuria is detected, a 24–h urine collection should be obtained. A renal biopsy is generally indicated if proteinuria is > 2.0 g qd, cellular casts are present or renal function is deteriorating (not otherwise explained). Some recommend the measurement of complement levels (which decrease when the disease is active) as a good indicator of renal disease activity, or an increase in ANA titers. Changes in complement levels and ANA titers can be nonspecific, however, and not always predictive of renal disease activity.

A renal biopsy helps to guide therapy in cases where clinical data is confusing or contradictory. Some clinicians argue that in a young patient with obvious active lupus, heavy proteinuria, and numerous red cell casts in the urine sediment, a renal biopsy is not necessary to confirm the presence of serious disease requiring aggressive therapy. If there is any diagnostic confusion, however, the renal biopsy will help the clinician to separate those with relatively benign lesions such as minimal change disease or focal segmental glomerulonephritis from those with more serious disease. More benign lesions may respond to corticosteroids alone or be observed, whereas membranoproliferative glomerulonephritis should be treated more aggressively, with cyclophosphamide and high-dose corticosteroids. Generally, more serious disease requires prednisone (prednisolone) 1mg kg/d for the first month, followed by a gradual taper to alternate day low-dose, and cyclophosphamide 750–1000 mg (15 mg/kg) is given every 3–4 weeks for at least 6 months to 1 year. There is controversy as to whether or not patients should remain on cyclophosphamide indefinitely (but receive doses at a reduced frequency), or be treated for 1–2 years and then observed.

Alternatives to cyclophosphamide include azathioprine, but this is probably less effective. The presence of an elevated creatinine level at the time of diagnosis of renal disease carries a worse prognosis, as does the finding of sclerosis and numerous crescents on biopsy. Lupus nephritis should be co-managed with a nephrologist and a rheumatologist.

Lupus cerebritis occurs in up to 15% of patients, manifesting as seizures, psychosis, stroke, delirium, transverse myelitis and, rarely, severe depression. Seizures are usually generalized, and are treated as one would any other type of seizure, but the occurrence suggests further immunosuppressive therapy is needed. There is no diagnostic test for lupus cerebritis as the cause for seizure or psychosis, but when these events occur, there is usually evidence of disease activity elsewhere (i.e. flare of rash or arthritis at the same time, or lymphopenia). One may also find focal neurologic findings suggestive of a stroke. Otherwise, one must rule out other causes (and examine cerebrospinal fluid) before attributing the patient's condition to lupus cerebritis. The treatment for cerebritis is controversial, doses of prednisone (prednisolone) 20–80 mg qd being recommended, tapering over several weeks to months with appropriate anti-seizure or anti-psychotic therapy as well. (One needs to differentiate lupus cerebritis from drug toxicity such as high-dose corticosteroids.) Cyclophospamide may be needed in severe cases, and is used as for renal disease. Transverse myelitis must be treated immediately to prevent paralysis.

Autoimmune hemolytic anemia or significant thrombocytopenia ($< 20\ 000 \times 10^9$/l, or clinical bleeding) is treated with high-dose prednisone (prednisolone) (60–80 mg qd), tapered over several weeks to months. Inability to withdraw corticosteroids after several weeks to months is an indication for considering danazol, other immunosuppressives, and splenectomy. Leukopenia does not need to be treated unless the WBC count is $< 2.0 \times 10^9$/l.

Raynaud's phenomenon is treated with nifedipine 20–40 mg qd (up to 80 mg qd if needed), or prazosin 1 mg bid. **One must recognize that many conditions may seem to mimic Raynaud's phenomenon. If not questioned properly, many patients will seem to experience it. Raynaud's phenomenon is the development of severe pallor of the digits followed by bluish discoloration, then erythema when it resolves. It is often (but not always) painful when it is red. Raynaud's phenomenon is not having cold feeling or aching in the digits when exposed to cold, having blue or purple discoloration first (must turn white first), having 'patches'** turning white when the skin is pressed, or having 'bad circulation and cold fingers all the time'. Raynaud's phenomenon never extends proximal to the MCP or MTP joints. To discover whether a patient has Raynaud's phenomenon, place their hands in a bowl of ice water, along with your own. Compare the color changes in the patient's hands with your own. This test is not 100% sensitive, but if what the patient's perceives to be 'colour changes' is reproduced, you can then know whether or not they are describing true Raynaud's phenomenon.

Patients with previous frostbite and whose occupation includes operating vibrating equipment may develop Raynaud's phenomenon, and so one should inquire about this prior to concluding they have SLE or scleroderma as the cause.

Lupus-like syndromes may be seen in patients taking procainamide (60% develop positive ANA in months with 20% developing SLE) and hydralazine (30% positive ANA and 10% SLE). These patients usually have polyarthritis and serositis, but not usually CNS or renal involvement, or anti-dsDNA antibodies. Although the ANA may persist for years, the symptoms resolve in months. Corticosteroids can be used for severe symptoms. Others responsible for lupus-like syndromes include isoniazid, chlorpromazine, penicillamine, methyldopa, minocycline oral contraceptives, phenytoin, and ethosuximide. Most lupus patients can be given these drugs safely, however.

Immunizations with influenza and pneumococcal vaccines are safe in controlled disease.

A summary of drug therapy of SLE is given in *Table 4.3*.

Laboratory findings

Serological findings include positive ANA, occasionally anti-dsDNA antibodies, false positive VDRL, and depressed serum complement. A negative ANA

Table 4.3 Summary of drug therapy of systemic lupus erythematosus

Manifestation	Therapy
Malar rash	Antimalarial (none if mild)
Discoid rash	Antimalarial ± topical corticosteroids ± intralesional corticosteroids
Photosensitivity	Antimalarial + sunscreens (Factor > 15)
Sjögren's syndrome	Artificial tears, frequent fluid intake, possibly antimalarial
Arthritis	Antimalarial, NSAIDs
Pneumonitis	NSAIDs or corticosteroids
Pericarditis	NSAIDs or corticosteroids
Lupus cerebritis	Corticosteroids ± cyclophosphamide
Hemolytic anemia	Corticosteroids
Nephritis	Corticosteroids ± cyclophosphamide ± azathioprine
Raynaud's phenomenon	Nifedipine, prazosin

virtually rules out the diagnosis since only rarely will rheumatologists diagnosis SLE with this negative finding. The patient may have hemolytic anemia, anemia of chronic disease, thrombocytopenia, leukopenia, and lymphopenia.

Hand X-rays will only rarely show bone erosions.

Case scenarios of SLE

1. *A 35-year-old woman with SLE is in remission on chloroquine 250 mg qd, and would like to have a planned pregnancy.* Make sure the patient understands the increased risk of spontaneous abortion, and the possibility of flare of the disease (usually post-partum). Pregnancy should not be considered until the disease activity is low or nonexistent clinically. (Some rheumatologists use other markers such as ANA titer levels being low.)

    Chloroquine is not available in the United States, and it is reported to have more ocular toxicity than hydroxychloroquine. Hydroxychloroquine is also used more frequently than chloroquine in the UK, although some rhematologists in both Canada and the UK continue to use chloroquine emphasizing that it is as effective, much less expensive, and that retinal toxicity is minimized by careful monitoring. The safety of chloroquine in pregnancy is documented by the large numbers of cases of anti-malarial prophylaxis in pregnant women. The safety of hydroxychloroquine in pregnancy is supported, to some extent, by studies in pregnant systemic lupus erythematosus patients.

    If the patient is against continuing an antimalarial, another option is prednisone 5–10 mg qd or alternate days to maintain disease remission, with the patient fully aware of adverse effects of systemic corticosteroids. This dose should be maintained post-partum for several weeks while the patient is restarted on an antimalarial, and the prednisone (prednisolone) tapered to discontinuation.

2. *A 35-year-old woman with SLE has delivered 2 days ago and now has developed arthritis, malar rash, hemoglobin of 4.0 × 10^9/l (normal = 12.0–16.0). She has also been noted to have 3+ proteinuria on dipstick, and red cell casts, with normal creatinine. She has been on no prior therapy.* The patient has had a post-partum flare of her disease. In most cases, where the flare is characterized by any of rash, arthritis, pleuritis, pericarditis, or neurologic events, therapy involves NSAIDs or systemic corticosteroids (e.g. prednisone (prednisolone) 30 mg po qd) depending on severity, and starting an anti-malarial if the patient has not been on one. In this case, however, there is a hemolytic anemia and nephritis. The hemolytic anemia is best treated with high-dose oral corticosteroids if there is no urgent need to give a transfusion. If there is, as in this case, high dose intravenous corticosteroids (e.g. methylprednisolone 1000 mg IV × 1) can be given. Blood can be transfused slowly (1 unit over 3–4 h), but no sooner than 6 h after

corticosteroid bolus. Without the time for corticosteroids to have their effect, transfusion will lead to further hemolysis, and possibly a hemolytic crisis with abdominal pain, hypotension, and even pulmonary edema.

NSAIDs should not be used if there is renal involvement. The patient should also have a 24–h urine collection and be seen by a nephrologist for renal biopsy when she is more stable. This will guide further therapy.

3. *A 55-year-old woman with SLE in remission on an antimalarial develops symptoms (chest pain, worse with inspiration), and signs (pericardial rub) of pericarditis.* Ask the patient about symptoms such as syncope or pre-syncope, dyspnea at rest or with exertion, and examine for elevated jugular venous pulse, and pulsus paradoxus. These suggest large effusions which may eventually require pericardiocentesis, and should prompt hospital admission with a visit from a cardiologist. The diagnosis can be confirmed by echocardiogram, but a more important reason for ordering this is to document the size of the pericardial effusion. If large, one should consider having the patient monitored in hospital.

One must rule out causes of pericarditis other than SLE. Viral pericarditis (hard to prove, and treated as for SLE pericarditis) may be preceded by an upper respiratory tract infection. Other considerations include uremia with pericarditis (check renal function and urinalysis), and rheumatic fever (Jones criteria). Therapy for SLE pericarditis is NSAIDs (e.g. indomethacin 50 mg po tid) or prednisone (prednisolone) 30 mg po qd for 3–4 weeks. If the patient is treated with NSAIDs and does not have symptomatic improvement in a few days, consider using corticosteroids. How long one should wait before considering corticosteroids depends on symptom severity. Milder symptoms mean the patient may be willing to wait longer for a response to the NSAID.

DOs and DON'Ts of Systemic Lupus Erythematosus (SLE)

DO use anti-malarial for the overall management of SLE.

DO have the patient seen by a rheumatologist.

DO advise against pregnancy when the disease is not controlled.

DO have a rheumatologist involved early if pregnancy is planned or has occurred.

DON'T diagnose Raynaud's phenomenon unless the patient gives a fairly classic history.

DON'T diagnose SLE on the basis of nondiagnostic symptoms and a positive ANA.

Section 4 – Localized pain and swelling

Seronegative spondyloarthropathy

When a patient presents with back pain that is worse when sitting or lying for long periods, and is improved by being active, consider a seronegative spondyloarthropathy. Mechanical back pain (see section on the painful back, page 146) may be worse with prolonged sitting or immobility, but is not clearly made better by becoming more active.

When a patient presents with back pain ask about morning stiffness (more than 1 hour is significant), pain that is less with activity than with rest, plantar fasciitis (a prolonged, days, episode of heel pain made worse with walking), iritis (an episode of marked eye pain, erythema, photophobia), conjunctivitis, psoriasis, urethral discharge or venereal disease, significant diarrheal illness, or bleeding per rectum. These are all clues to the seronegative spondyloarthropathies.

Algorithmic Approach

When a patient presents with back pain typical of spondylitis, the diagnosis is simpler than if they present with arthritis alone. The algorithm will help to sort the latter out, however.

The patient complains of localized pain, with or without back pain, so you are traveling down the left side of the algorithm. The patient complains of joint swelling. If it is one joint, then one must consider whether or not the attack is brief or prolonged. The possibilities are: palindromic arthritis; crystal arthropathy; septic arthritis; or spondyloarthropathy.

Spondyloarthropathy of one joint is considered when an episode is prolonged, as stated in the algorithm. The separation of the above is by joint aspiration and reviewing the diagnostic criteria for spondyloarthropathy:

Nocturnal pain or morning stiffness of lumbar or dorsal spine?	Yes
Asymmetric arthritis?	Yes
Alternating right and left buttock pain?	No

Sausage digit?	No
Plantar fasciitis?	Yes
Iritis?	No
One of psoriasis, balanitis, or inflammatory bowel disease	Yes, psoriasis
Positive family history?	No
HLA-B27 positive?	This test is not required

So the patient has psoriatic arthritis. The different types of spondylo-arthropathy are included in this list, and so one immediately has an easy way of knowing that a patient with arthritis could have any of ankylosing spondylitis, psoriatic arthritis, reactive arthritis, or bowel-associated arthritis: the reminders are each in the above list of questions. If this approach is taken with each patient with polyarticular arthritis, a spondylo-arthropathy will not be missed.

The seronegative spondyloarthropathies lack an association with rheumatoid factor and have in common a high frequency of HLA-B27 positivity, iritis, spine and sacroiliac disease, and a variable extent of peripheral arthritis. This group contains ankylosing spondylitis, psoriatic arthritis, reactive arthritis (including Reiter's syndrome), and bowel-associated arthritis. Bowel-associated arthritis (or enteropathic arthritis) has similar features to the seronegative spondyloarthropathies, but is not HLA-B27 associated. The different types are distinguished from each other by certain clinical manifestations or disease associations, although at times it may be difficult to classify the patient from the outset.

An enthesopathy is responsible for many of the features. It involves inflammation, fibrosis, and ossification (reactive bone formation) at the enthesis (site of insertion of ligaments, tendons, and joint capsules to bone). In the spine, this causes destruction of the outer insertion sites of the disc annulus fibrosus to the vertebra (causing 'squaring' of the vertebra), vertebral end-plate destruction (causing apparent narrowing of the disc space), syndesmophytes as a result of reactive bone formation (linking the vertebrae), and reactive bone formation at the capsule insertion sites of the facet joints. The end result is ankylosis of these joints, and a 'stiff' spine. The enthesopathy at ligamentous fibers between the sacral and iliac bones, as well as inflammation within the synovial, inferior aspect of the sacroiliac joint leads to bone sclerosis, then ossification and ankylosis of that joint as well. Many other sites of enthesitis occur, such as at the insertion of the plantar fascia and Achilles tendon to the calcaneus, the capsular insertions of the costovertebral, sternoclavicular, sternomanubrial, and costochondral joints, the capsules and ligaments around finger joints, and tendon sheaths (producing dactylitis or 'sausage digits').

Ankylosing spondylitis

Ankylosing spondylitis refers to the primary form of sacroiliitis, that is in the absence of features that suggest one of the other seronegative spondylo-arthropathies, or other causes of sacroiliitis (osteoarthritis, gout, bacterial infection, tuberculosis, brucellosis). It typically occurs in young men.

Examination of the spine may reveal restriction of movement in all directions (but not always in early or mild disease), a positive modified Schober's test (mark the level of the posterior iliac spines, sacral dimples, and a point 10 cm above this in the spinal midline. When the patient flexes the spine forward, the distance between the two points increases to at least 15 cm in normal subjects), and muscle spasm. Upper spine involvement is documented by the 'occiput-wall' test. (In the normal subject, when the heels, buttocks, and scapulae are against the wall, the occiput also makes contact with the wall when the head is upright. In ankylosing spondylitis there is a distance separating the occiput from the wall.) In advanced disease, dorsal spine involvement is evidenced by loss of lateral rotation and chest expansion (normal > 5 cm at the level of the axillae). A neurologic deficit is usually not found but may occur late in the disease, as a cauda equina syndrome. Spine fractures may occur with minimal trauma.

See *Figures 4.1–4.7* below for the specific examination techniques in suspected ankylosing spondylitis.

One must distinguish the much more common 'mechanical' back pain from true sacroiliitis. Patients with mechanical back pain have worse pain with activity than with rest (the reverse is generally true in sacroiliitis). Mechanical back pain may produce morning stiffness, although it is usually not prolonged. Unlike patients with sacroiliitis, patients with mechanical back pain usually have pain with hyperextension. Patients with mechanical back pain tend to have palpable tenderness over the muscles of the lumbosacral region and gluteal muscles, which is extremely uncommon in sacroiliitis.

So-called sacroiliac 'stress' maneuvers are usually negative in sacroiliitis. These include pelvic compression by applying simultaneous lateral, inward pelvic pressure, hyperextension of one limb off the examining table while the patient is supine, and externally rotating the hip while it is in abduction and flexion. These tests are often positive in some patients with mechanical back pain. See the section on the painful back (page 146) for further discussion on how to distinguish ankylosing spondylitis clinically from mechanical back pain.

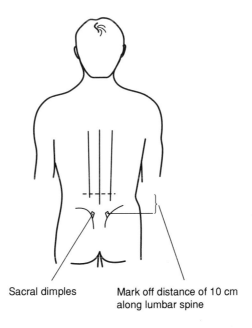

Sacral dimples   Mark off distance of 10 cm
                        along lumbar spine

Fig. 4.1   Modified Schrober test to detect restricted lumbar flexion.

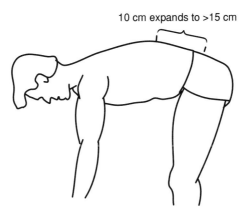

10 cm expands to >15 cm

Fig. 4.2   Profile of forward lumbar flexion.

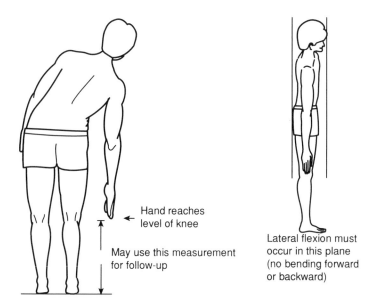

Hand reaches
level of knee

May use this measurement
for follow-up

Lateral flexion must
occur in this plane
(no bending forward
or backward)

Fig. 4.3 Lateral lumbar flexion.

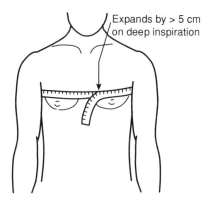

Expands by > 5 cm
on deep inspiration

Fig. 4.4 Measuring chest expansion. (Measure circumference at nipple line.)

Enthesopathy elsewhere may produce pleuritic chest pain (e.g. costochondral joints), heel pain with burning on the sole of the foot (plantar fascia), and dactylitis. A peripheral arthritis involving usually large joints may occur, and has inflammatory characteristics on synovial fluid analysis. The arthritis may precede or follow spine disease by years.

Iritis occurs in 20–40% of cases and has little correlation with the spine disease, occurring years before or after. Symptoms are treated with indomethacin, topical corticosteroids, or sometimes systemic corticosteroids.

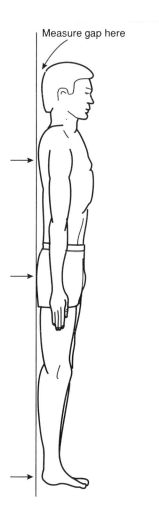

Measure gap here

Fig. 4.5 Measuring wall–occiput distance.

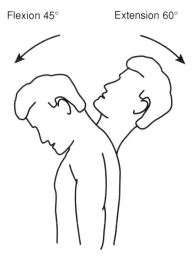

Flexion 45°   Extension 60°

Fig. 4.6 Neck flexion and extension.

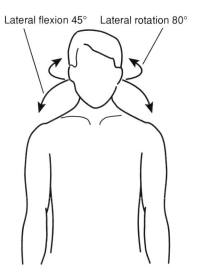

Lateral flexion 45°   Lateral rotation 80°

Fig. 4.7 Neck lateral flexion and rotation.

Prompt recognition and treatment is important, and an ophthalmologic opinion is worthwhile.

Other disease complications include interstitial lung disease with fibrosis and occasionally cavitation in upper lobes, restrictive lung disease due to spine fusion, aortic regurgitation, and atrioventricular conduction defects.

Radiological diagnosis is made via a simple anteroposterior view of the pelvis. The findings may progress from initial widening of the sacroiliac joint (during bone destruction), then bony sclerosis (bone formation) on both sides of the joint, with narrowing and bridging of the bone across the joint, and possibly eventual fusion. Primary sacroiliitis (ankylosing spondylitis) tends to produce symmetric involvement, whereas the other spondyloarthropathies tend to produce asymmetric or even unilateral involvement. If the inferior margins of the sacroiliac joint are spared, one should suspect osteoarthritis or infection rather than spondyloarthropathy. Also, osteophytes of the spine from osteoarthritis tend to be more horizontal whereas in spondyloarthropathies the syndesmophytes are more vertical, and usually larger.

Early in the disease (< 6 months), the X-rays may be normal. At this stage, a bone scan or a CT scan may be positive and should be ordered if the diagnosis is still suspected.

The treatment is indomethacin, sometimes requiring up to 200 mg qd initially, tapering the dose to as low as tolerable for maintenance. Other NSAIDs are also effective. Sulfasalazine may be of benefit. Some patients may require agents such as methotrexate, as used in rheumatoid arthritis (usually a rheumatologist should be involved at this point). Some sites of enthesopathy may be treated with corticosteroid injection. It is controversial as to whether or not a patient whose back symptoms have remitted and who is on an exercise program should continue to use indomethacin, for example. Some argue that the enthesitis responsible for the disease should be kept entirely inactive so as to prevent bony ankylosis of the spine. A maintenance dose of 50 mg qd or a few times per week may be sufficient. Others argue that the cost and adverse effects of the NSAID do not warrant this approach, but rather that the patient should only use the NSAID when symptomatic.

It is believed that if an individual has had symptoms of ankylosing spondylitis for 10 years, but has not yet had spine fusion, he or she is unlikely to develop spine fusion after that time.

An exercise regimen is extremely important, and includes twice daily spine extension exercises. Good posture should be trained, and the patient should have a firm mattress.

Reactive arthritis and Reiter's syndrome

Reactive arthritis is a seronegative spondyloarthropathy that is thought to occur following exposure to an infectious agent which induces an immunologic response culminating in arthritis, mucositis, enthesopathy, and ocular disease. The infection is not active within the joints, however, and so it is not a septic arthritis. Reiter's syndrome is one type of reactive arthritis in which certain classic extra-articular features are seen. These are typically not seen in the other seronegative spondyloarthropathies. Reiter's syndrome is called 'post-dysenteric' following infections with *Shigella flexneri*, *Salmonella* species, *Yersinia* species, and *Campylobacter* species, and 'post-venereal' Reiter's following infections with *Chlamydia* species and *Ureaplasma urealyticum*. Reiter's syndrome is also seen in AIDS.

A variety of other infections are associated with arthritis, but lack the immunologic (e.g. HLA-B27) and disease (e.g. psoriasis) associations seen in the seronegative spondyloarthropathies. These infections include arthritis following bacterial infection (but not septic arthritis), spirochetes as in syphilis and Lyme disease, mycobacterial, viral, and parasitic infections. Note that post-gonococcal arthritis is considered a septic arthritis, not specifically a reactive arthritis.

Reactive arthritis has the features (clinical, laboratory, and radiological) common to seronegative spondyloarthropathies. The onset may be insidious or acute, with fever and fatigue or weight loss. The arthritis is usually oligoarticular, but may be polyarticular.

The classic triad of Reiter's syndrome is arthritis, urethritis, and conjunctivitis. Typically, however, most cases lack one or two of these features. The associated infection may occur up to 1 month prior to onset of the arthritis, and the patient may not have symptoms of that infection at the time when arthritis appears, or the infection may have been asymptomatic to begin with. Other findings include oral and genital (e.g. balanitis) inflammatory lesions, which are usually asymptomatic. They are erythematous, painless, and discrete. The patient with post-venereal Reiter's may develop inflammatory lesions of the gut mucosa, and therefore diarrhea, confusing the issue as to which type of infection (venereal or dysenteric) is responsible. The reverse is also possible. On the skin, an inflammatory lesion indistinguishable from pustular psoriasis occurs on the palms and soles (keratoderma blenorrhagicum), and hyperkeratosis of the nails is diagnostic.

Reactive arthritis can only be diagnosed when the individual either has classic findings of Reiter's syndrome, or has a clear history of an antecedent infection. Also, the patient will not have psoriasis. Otherwise, there are no specific diagnostic tests.

Therapy is as for ankylosing spondylitis. Some believe it is also important, where possible, to treat the patient with antibiotics directed at the original infection, for example doxycycline 250 mg bid for 4–6 weeks.

Chronic diarrhea is not a finding in reactive arthritis, so one should suspect inflammatory bowel disease if this occurs.

Psoriatic arthritis

Psoriasis is associated with a seronegative spondyloarthropathy, and the peripheral arthritis may be the most prominent feature. The skin manifestations may precede or follow the arthritis by many years. There is poor correlation between the severity of the skin lesions and the arthritis. The clinical manifestations include those common to all seronegative spondyloarthropathies. A severe form of psoriasis and arthritis can occur in HIV-positive patients.

The arthritis may be oligoarticular, affecting the DIP, PIP, MCP, MTP, hip, or knee joints, or polyarticular (sometimes symmetric and mimicking rheumatoid arthritis). The sacroilitis tends to be mild and asymmetric. Arthritis mutilans is a severe destructive form in which osteolysis of the phalangeal and metacarpal or metatarsal bones occurs.

Psoriasis is a papulosquamous, coarse scaling lesion. It may be localized (scalp, chest, periumbilicus, perianal, and extensor limb surfaces), may have accompanying pustular lesions, diffuse erythroderma, and generalized exfoliative dermatitis. Nail changes associated with psoriasis include pitting, onycholysis with discoloration of the nail edge, subungual hyperkeratosis, and transverse ridges. These changes may be present in the absence of psoriasis skin lesions. Normal subjects may have nail pits, but the presence of 20 pits in total suggests psoriatic arthritis, more than 60 being diagnostic.

Radiographs reveal an erosive arthritis that may mimic rheumatoid arthritis, but important differentiating features are asymmetry, relative absence of the periarticular osteopenia seen in rheumatoid arthritis, and predominant involvement of the DIP joints with osteolysis of the terminal phalanges. Asymmetric sacroiliitis, and atypical (asymmetric, few in number) syndesmophytes may also be seen.

If NSAIDs fail, antimalarials, sulfasalazine, gold, penicillamine, and methotrexate in doses used for rheumatoid arthritis can be used in psoriatic arthritis. The use of the antimalarials is controversial since some believe they may produce increased episodes of exfoliative reactions. (Hydroxychloroquine is believed to be less likely to do this.) Methotrexate is particularly effective in managing the skin disease as well. Systemic corticosteroids should not be used since tapering tends to cause an exacerbation of the skin disease. The skin disease is treated with topical preparations of tar, dithranol, and corticosteroids, as well as vitamin D and ultraviolet light therapy. Co-management with a dermatologist is recommended if the skin disease is significant or difficult to control.

Bowel-associated (enteropathic) arthritis

Enteropathic arthritis should be distinguished from the association of seronegative spondyloarthropathies with various forms of gastrointestinal disease. Reiter's syndrome following an infectious enteritis is one example of this association. Bowel-associated or enteropathic arthritis, however, is not HLA-B27 associated, and is seen in association with inflammatory bowel disease and intestinal bypass.

It occurs in 10–20% of patients with Crohn's disease or ulcerative colitis. The peripheral arthritis activity parallels the bowel disease activity, but the spinal component may not correlate with the bowel disease, sometimes progressing despite adequate therapy for the bowel inflammation. Removal of the colon in ulcerative colitis clearly alters the course of the peripheral arthritis, but not the axial involvement.

Treatment involves sulfasalazine (for both bowel and joints). Additionally NSAIDs or drugs such as methotrexate are sometimes needed. The long held concern that gold could worsen the patient's colitis may be unsubstantiated, but NSAIDs may do so.

The disease following small bowel bypass used in treating morbid obesity is characterized by polyarthritis and rarely spine disease. Patients commonly have a papulovesicular or urticarial, macular rash. The arthritis is treated as above, but is also ameliorated by reanastomosis of the bypassed bowel. It is less common these days because the surgery is used less often.

DOs and DON'Ts of Seronegative Spondyloarthropathies

DO consider ankylosing spondylitis in any patient with marked morning stiffness (more than 1 h) who prefers NOT to rest when back pain is severe, but would rather stretch or remain active.

DO realize that even patients with mechanical back pain may complain of morning stiffness, but it usually is of much shorter duration.

DO ask patients with back pain about symptoms of iritis (severe eye pain, erythema, tearing, photophobia), plantar fascitis (marked heel pain, worst first thing in the morning when walking), psoriasis, spontaneous acute swelling of one whole digit, symptoms of inflammatory bowel disease (bloody diarrhea), urethral discharge, recent venereal disease or significant diarrheal illness. These are seen in seronegative spondyloarthropathy.

DO remember that patients with ankylosing spondylitis are tender over the spinous processes, but generally not elsewhere (as is the case with mecahanical or myofascial back pain).

DO consider seronegative spondyloarthropathy when a young patient has recurrent or persistent swelling of lower limb joints, without much upper limb involvement, and no evidence of crystals in joint fluid.

Section 5 –
Outside the algorithm

Other conditions

There are a number of rheumatic diseases and conditions which are not shown in the algorithm, chiefly because they are not typically presenting with joint pain or stiffness. The following sections will deal with back pain, neck pain, scleroderma, polymyositis, vasculitis, and reflex sympathetic dystrophy. These are all far less common than chronic pain syndromes, tendinitis, and arthritis, but one can still be alerted to them by specific presenting complaints. Thus each of the following sections will be introduced with 'When a patient has x, consider y'.

Section 5 – Outside the algorithm

> # Painful
> # back

Back pain is discussed here for convenience while we are on the subject of regional pain.

The management of back pain can be approached with a variety of philosophies. The following discussion gives an idea of how most rheumatologists approach back pain in the patients commonly seen in rheumatology clinics. From the start, it should be mentioned that the author agrees with and recommends the text *The Back Doctor* by Dr Hamilton Hall (McClelland-Bantam Inc., Toronto, 1980), to be read by physicians and patients.

Rheumatologists tend to classify most cases of back pain as 'mechanical back pain'. By this, they are acknowledging a somewhat limited understanding of how the many structures of the back and pelvis, including ligaments, muscles, fascia, bursa, facet joints, vertebral discs, and sacroiliac joints may be affected or act to produce pain. Rheumatologists do recognize four common patterns of back pain, however, and can assess and manage back pain on this basis rather than focus on anatomic diagnoses.

Some practitioners are quite confident that they can identify the exact structure or mechanism responsible for the patient's pain. Thus, terms such as 'L3–L4 dislocation', 'sacroiliac dysfunction or dislocation', 'malalignment of the spine', etc., are used by some. Most rheumatologists would classify all these 'different' disorders as mechanical back pain. The author will not defend or invalidate either of these philosophies, but will simply describe the one held by most rheumatologists.

Mechanical back pain may originate from key structures such as the facet joints (the posterior articulation of one vertebra with those above and below), the vertebral discs, and impingement of spinal nerves. This is not to say that other structures are not important, nor are we sure how these structures cause the pain. Years from now we may find our current concepts to be incorrect.

What is observed quite reproducibly is that patients with mechanical back pain tend to have similar symptoms, aggravating factors, and natural history. When a patient complains of back pain, it is worthwhile to ask whether or not they have pain elsewhere, as they may have a chronic pain syndrome.

After this, the key questions to ask deal with whether or not there are features which make one concerned the patient has pain due to something other than mechanical back pain, and then if these are not present, distinguishing mechanical back pain from spondylitis.

One may proceed as follows.

1. Although realizing that mechanical back pain is the most common form, one would like to affirm that other causes are not present. Start then with asking about nocturnal onset of pain without day-time pain, weight loss, fever, bladder or bowel incontinence (except stress incontinence), fixed or progressive objective neurologic deficit (like drop foot or leg weakness), and known history of malignancy.

   If these are present, then one must order X-rays, CT or MRI scans, bone scans, etc. Mechanical back pain will actually be the end-result in some of these cases, but they must all be investigated if these warning signs are present.

   Then ask about the circumstances in which pain occurs. Pain which is worse on activity is more likely to be mechanical in origin. Pain that improves with activity is more likely to be spondylitis. Pain that is neither, that is, not seemingly related by the patient to be worsened or improved by activity is of more concern (including possibilities such as malignancy, and pain from an intra-abdominal or intra-thoracic origin). Mechanical back pain is made worse towards the end of the active (or working) period or day. When one asks what the patient does at a time when the pain is at its worst, the patient with mechanical back pain will almost always say rest in some fashion. Recall in the section on ankylosing spondylitis, that a patient with sacroiliitis will tend to continue activity when the pain is bad, since not doing so causes more stiffness and pain.

   Ask the patient about pain when attempting to get in and out of a car, or using a vacuum cleaner. Aggravating factors of 'activity', 'flexion', or 'extension' are specific enough to diagnose mechanical back pain. Considering further the specific questions about the circumstances of pain, recognize that there are four chief patterns of mechanical pain, and listen for them, as they will confirm your suspicions.

   Pattern 1.   The pain is mostly in the back, worse with flexion or sitting for long periods, pain attacks gradually developing over hours to days, and present for weeks to months.
   Pattern 2.   The pain is mostly in the back, worse with extension (getting up from a flexed posture), often attacks are of sudden onset (minutes to hours) and last for days to weeks.
   Pattern 3.   The pain is mostly in the lower limb, worse with flexion or sitting for long periods, pain attacks gradually developing over hours to days, lasting weeks to months.

Pattern 4. The pain is mostly in the lower limb. It begins when standing, or shortly after standing, becomes worse with walking, and is relieved in 5–10 minutes by changing from standing to sitting after walking. This is spinal claudication.

Pattern 5. The pain is severe, diffuse, present every day, and accompanied by many of the symptoms (when inquired about) typical of chronic pain syndromes. (See the section on chronic pain syndromes, page 26)

Patients whose pain is worst with flexion may have disc disease, those with pain on extension may have facet joint disease, and those with spinal claudication may have spinal stenosis. Patterns may co-exist. Ask the patient not where all their pain is (it may be in many sites), but rather whether their pain is predominantly in the back or the legs. This will allow you to identify one of the four mechanical patterns above.

Acute disc protrusion is characterized by acute onset of back pain followed by radicular pain, and numbness in the lower limb. Often, specific signs of nerve root compression are evident: sensory loss in medial calf (L4), lateral calf (L5), lateral foot (S1), weakness of dorsiflexion (L5) or plantar flexion (S1), and reduced knee (L4) or ankle (L5) reflexes.

2. Ask about stiffness. Stiffness first thing in the morning is seen in both mechanical back pain and spondylitis. The difference is that any period of immobility worsens the stiffness of spondylitis, like lying down during the day, and the morning stiffness lasts longer than in mechanical back pain (usually the latter is relieved within 15 min). The patient with mechanical back pain will describe being in a stooped posture in the morning, with pain when trying to straighten up, but again this is short-lived.

3. Realize that mechanical back pain may be of gradual or acute onset, so this is not a useful diagnostic clue. As well, the pain may be felt across the low back, gluteals, and radiate to the feet in a variety of directions. There is little diagnostic value in knowing exactly which contortion causes the back pain, although patients often think such details are very important.

Amount of pain is not relevant to outcome. Overwhelming pain is not necessarily indicative of a more serious disease, and does not necessitate investigations any more than a patient with less pain.

You will now have enough information to proceed with examination. The patient who has the worrisome type of back pain as described above will have a complete examination, looking for some malignancy in most cases. The remainder will be determined by examination of the back in a specific manner.

Examination of the lumbar spine

This may seem to be a overly simple method, but it actually suffices for most patients.

1. Examine the gait and posture. In mechanical back pain, there will be a normal gait when the pain is not acute, since otherwise the patient may have a flexed posture, or if they have a true nerve impingement (which can be confirmed by neurologic examination) their gait may be abnormal due to weakness of one leg. A chronic flexed posture can only be due to vertebral body collapse and subsequent kyphosis, ankylosing spondylitis, or malingering.

2. Ask the patient to bend forwards to touch their toes without bending their knees, and then ask them to stand up straight. The majority of patients with chronic mechanical back pain have near normal range of flexion, but will often say that pain occurs during forward flexion, with a 'pulling sensation.' The same will occur with lateral flexion. They will also find that they have pain when standing up from the flexed posture, again typical of mechanical back pain. Hyperextension (that is, actually having the patient bend backward as far as they can (arching their back while standing) is also often uncomfortable in mechanical back pain.

   The range of flexion is useful. Most patients with chronic mechanical back pain actually can flex to get their fingertips within 20 cm of the floor. If they cannot, they either have an acute episode, are malingering, have a chronic pain syndrome, or ankylosing spondylitis. The diagnosis of ankylosing spondylitis depends on finding other symptoms and signs (see the section on seronegative spondyloarthropathy, page 133).

   Signs of 'nonstructural' back pain which may represent chronic pain syndrome, or a tendency to exaggerate pain:
   (a) With the patient standing, touch the skin of the low back lightly, or gently squeeze the skin of the lower back between your fingers.
   (b) With the patient standing, apply downward pressure on the top of the head.
   (c) Ask the patient to kneel and then sit with their legs flexed underneath them. Ask the patient to try to bend forwards in this position (*Figure 5.1*).

Pain with these maneuvers indicates a tendency to exaggerate pain or a significant psychological influence over pain.

   For signs of malingering:
   (a) If the patient has a limp, ask them to walk forwards and backwards and see if the limp changes (it shouldn't).
   (b) With the patient supine, flex their hip to 90°, with the knee flexed at

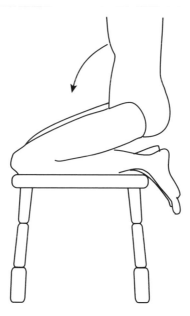

Fig. 5.1 A test for malingering or chronic pain syndrome. (The chief movement is in the hip joint, not the spine.)

90°. Rotate the hip joint 30° in either direction. Back pain should not occur unless the patient is malingering.

(c) Have the patient dorsiflex at the ankle joint, and resist this flexion. In true weakness, the foot gives way smoothly. In others the ankle dorsiflexion gives way in a 'cogwheel' (a little at a time) effect instead.

(d) With the patient supine, do a straight leg raise, and note at what angle pain is felt. Then have the patient sit with their legs hanging off the examining table. Now extend the knee fully. In true nerve root irritation, pain will occur with both straight leg raising, and extending the knee in the seated position. If it occurs with straight leg raising only, malingering is likely.

(e) With the patient supine, do the straight leg raise with one leg and note the angle at which it becomes painful. Then repeat the raise, but with both legs at the same time. Normally this should lead to less pain at the angle that was previously painful. If pain occurs at a lower angle than with the single leg raise, malingering is likely.

(f) If the patient demonstrates a sensory loss in the limb to pinprick or touch, use a tuning fork to test vibration in that region. Place the tuning fork over a bony prominence in the region, and ask the patient if they can feel vibration anywhere. If they state they cannot feel vibration anywhere, there are only three possibilities: malingering; widespread neuropathy of that limb; or stocking distribution vibration loss as seen in diabetes. The reason is that vibration is normally conducted from one bone to others in a limb, so that a patient with true sensory loss on examination in the S1 distribution only, for instance, will have vibration loss over the lateral malleolus, but will feel the vibration conducted to the medial malleolus (a different dermatome). The only way they could not is if they have a neuropathy affecting the region of the medial malleolus as well. (But the sensory loss to pinprick or touch was only demonstrated for S1, so this could not be the case.)

3. With the patient lying on their abdomen, mechanical back pain is associated with tenderness not only over the spinous processes, but also when a forceful downward thrust towards the examining table is made with the thumbs applied just above the buttocks and lateral to the spine itself (this produces a sudden hyperextension in a sense). Beyond noting this finding, detailed palpation for exact location of tenderness in the back is not very useful in adding to the diagnostic capability. Patients with mechanical back pain tend to have a number of tender sites in the low back region and gluteal muscles. It is quite uncommon for a patient with ankylosing spondylitis to have this form of tenderness. In fact, if a patient is complaining of low back or gluteal pain, and one cannot find tenderness there, the patient has either referred pain (i.e. intra-abdominal organ, aortic aneurysm, renal infection) or ankylosing spondylitis. Patients with ankylosing spondylitis do not have areas of tenderness over one part of the spine, say T6–T9, and then no tenderness until L1–L4. Ankylosing spondylitis does not 'skip' regions like this, but mechanical back pain commonly does.

If the patient has marked tenderness over just the spinous processes of 1–3 vertebra and nowhere else in the back, then an X-ray of that region is warranted.

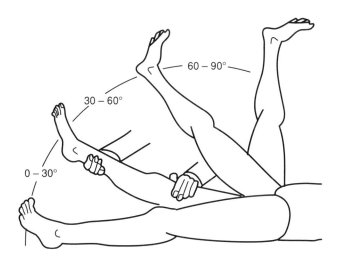

60 – 90°

30 – 60°

0 – 30°

Fig. 5.2 Straight leg raising as a positive sign.

4. Next do straight leg raising. This is commonly painful in mechanical back pain. It is rare for straight leg raising to be painful at less than 30° in disc protrusion. If so, it represents a disc protrusion that is also causing an objective neurologic deficit (like abnormal reflexes) or, more usually it represents a chronic pain syndrome or malingering. Pain with straight leg raising at 30–60° is often correlated with disc protrusion, but pain after 60° can be found in many causes of back pain, and therefore one has to look at other parts of the examination (*Figure 5.2*).

5. The neurologic examination helps to rule out nerve impingement or more serious spinal cord pathology. Strength and reflexes should be normal if there is no nerve impingement, although the sensation is commonly altered in mechanical back pain in distributions that do not conform to dermatomes. In the absence of abnormal reflexes or muscle weakness, this is not concerning. The peripheral pulses should be checked, and in older patients one should examine for abdominal bruits.

6. If the history suggests spondylitis, and the above examination is not typical of mechanical back pain, measure the lumbar flexion, chest expansion, and wall-occiput distance as described in the section on seronegative spondyloarthropathy (page 133).

Key examination points
- Are you examining a patient who actually has a chronic pain syndrome, but is merely focusing on this one of many sites of pain today?
- Exact localization of the spot on the back that is painful is not helpful.
- Sacroiliac stress tests are regarded by many to be useless.
- Positive straight leg raising after 60° may occur in many forms of back pain.

One should now have distinguished between mechanical back pain, spondylitis, malingering, or chronic pain syndrome. If spondylitis is suspected on the basis of the history and examination, then anteroposterior X-ray of the pelvis, and bone scan are useful (although some physicians use CT scans as well). See the section on seronegative spondyloarthropathy (page 133).

The last pattern of mechanical back pain – spinal claudication – may be due to spinal stenosis. Patients describe back pain which occurs usually with walking short distances (< 300 m), that becomes relieved within minutes if they change their posture to more flexion, sitting or lying, but not if they simply stand still (standing still tends to relieve vascular claudication). The pain of spinal claudication tends to begin in the back and radiate to the legs, whereas vascular claudication is usually the reverse. Some may describe foot drop as they walk (their toe tends to catch or drag as they are walking). Patients may have significant abnormalities on X-ray, but have no symptoms. On the other hand, they may have mild X-ray changes and yet be found on CT scan or other imaging to have spinal stenosis. If a young patient develops such symptoms, other imaging is definitely required even if the X-rays are normal, since young patients may have a spinal cord mass responsible for their stenosis. Remember, however, that the finding of spinal stenosis on a CT or MRI scan does not make the diagnosis of spinal claudication. The patient must give a clear history of spinal claudication as well. Otherwise the finding on the scan of spinal stenosis is incidental and does not require surgical intervention.

X-rays are for the most part not needed to diagnose or treat mechanical back pain. They are most often ordered to alleviate any worry on the physician's part of something more serious (like a vertebral fracture in a young person with no history of trauma), to make the patient feel they are being completely assessed, and in older patients to look for vertebral fractures, which may or may not alter therapy. One approach to conserve expense is to treat the mechanical back pain for at least 6–8 weeks, and only do an X-ray if the patient has not improved at all, but appears to be following your advice. There is little correlation between the X-ray findings and the patient's symptoms.

One should not order CT scans, myelograms, or MRI scans on patients with back pain unless the history strongly suggests some disorder like a disc protrusion, or spinal claudication, or an ominous disease (weight loss, fever, nocturnal pain only, etc.). Otherwise, sending patients with chronic pain syndromes or nonspecific mechanical back pain or chronic back pain after an accident will inevitably coincide with some finding on CT scan which prompts inappropriate referrals or surgery, even though it is not responsible for the pain.

CT and MRI scans may find anatomic abnormalities whose significance and natural history are not fully known. One should be looking for something specific when ordering these scans. If every patient with back pain had a scan, abnormalities would indeed be found in a number, but the majority would be of no clinical significance.

Management

The treatment for chronic back pain recommended by many rheumatologists is exercise and improvement in posture. (See Appendix 5 and *The Back Doctor*). These exercises can be taught to the patient by the physician or a physiotherapist. The patient should not be returning to the physiotherapist regularly, but should be doing the exercises at home; it is their responsibility to do these exercises if they want to improve their pain. Dependency on the physician or physiotherapist is counterproductive.

Very often these patients do not respond dramatically to chronic analgesics or NSAIDs for pain, and such therapies, by themselves, do not actually alter the underlying problem. Some recommend corticosteroid injections at trigger or tender points or near specific structures. Others do not believe these to be helpful, and treat back pain quite successfully without them.

It is important to tell patients with mechanical back pain that they will not become paralyzed or permanently disabled, and will not develop crippling arthritis of the spine. Mechanical back pain should be a rare cause for a disability pension. Patients should return to work entirely if they do their exercises. They must be told that they will have back pain when they return to work, but pain without neurologic deficit is not a reason to stop working. One should not use absence of pain as an indication of readiness for work. Most patients would never return to work if this was the case. They do not actually benefit (relief from back pain) in the long term from stopping work.

For very acute mechanical back pain, many recommend rest for the first 1–3 days. At this point many treatment regimens can be attempted. Patients and practitioners will seek out various aids such as medications (analgesics or NSAIDs), back manipulation, corticosteroid injections, ultrasound, heat, ice, etc. Many of these help some patients quite well, but the efficacy of each is variable. The patient should realize that analgesics in this period are being used to reduce the suffering associated with the normal resolution of acute back pain. Such therapy will not treat the actual problem. Only early mobilization, and return to prescribed exercises will help do this.

After the first 1–3 days of rest, patients can do some relatively harmless exercises while waiting for their back pain to settle. These include simply tightening the stomach muscles with the knees bent. After the rest period, the patient should be encouraged to walk about the house and take part in daily activities of living as much as possible, not to lie in bed constantly. The patient must realize that as they begin to walk and move about the house, that they will have pain, but one should not consider this pain to be an omen of relapse, and it should not lead to an immediate return to bed rest. Patients should avoid any lifting, avoid sitting for long periods (eat standing up until things improve), and when lying on their back, do so with a pillow under their knees, or on their side with a pillow between their knees.

Acute disc protrusion causing nerve impingement is treated no differently at the onset. The patient should be given the same advice as above, but the exercise regimen is not used. Instead, these patients are given adequate NSAIDs to control their pain, and their symptoms are followed. They will be able to (in a few days) walk with mild discomfort. How long someone with a nerve impingement should wait with conservative therapy before considering surgical therapy is debatable. A progressive neurologic deficit despite rest and NSAIDs, for example, is an indication for radiologic assessment (CT scan/myelogram) and referral to a surgeon. When one observes the typical history and physical findings of an acute disc protrusion with nerve impingement, the diagnosis does not need radiologic confirmation. When there are bilateral neurologic deficits, or if they are progressive, or the patient has other symptoms (e.g. fever), then the need for further investigations and referral exists. Many surgeons use 3–6 months of conservative therapy with little or no improvement, before surgery is done. Bladder or bowel incontinence warrants surgical referral. Less than 2% of all patients with back pain will ever need surgery.

Some patients with spinal stenosis improve with abdominal strengthening exercises, NSAIDs, or epidural saline or corticosteroid injections. Others will need spinal decompression to treat their symptoms.

DOs and DON'Ts of Back Pain

DO ask about weight loss, fever, bladder or bowel incontinence, and nocturnal onset of back pain. Some of these patients will have diseases other than mechanical back pain.

DO look for one of the four patterns of mechanical back pain and explain to the patient that these are common, nondisabling back disorders, that respond well to exercises if the patient makes the effort.

DO explain to the patient that readiness to return to work is not determined by lack of pain. They will have pain when they return to work, but will never damage their back from doing so. At most, a patient may take a few weeks off work to start an exercise program.

DO refer the patient to an exercise-oriented clinic that encourages independent therapy and early return to work.

DON'T tell the patient they will have a progressive arthritis of the spine. They will not, but if enough people tell them so a chronic pain syndrome will develop.

DON'T routinely order X-rays. Explain to the patient that X-rays are not needed at this time, but will be considered only if symptoms persist or worsen despite the patient's attempts at appropriate exercises.

DON'T order CT or MRI scans unless one has clear, objective clinical findings suggestive of disc protrusion with neurologic deficit or spinal claudication. Pain is not an indication for these scans, no matter how severe.

DON'T let patients become obsessed with X-ray findings.

DON'T treat chronic mechanical back pain with narcotics.

DON'T prescribe corsets for back pain.

DON'T allow the patient to become dependent on regular physiotherapy

---

Section 5 – Outside the algorithm

> # Painful
> # neck

Virtually all cases of neck pain are chronic pain syndromes or mechanical neck pain.

When a patient complains of neck pain, the first step is to determine whether or not they also have pain in their arms, chest, lower back, etc., as they probably then have a chronic pain syndrome. The whole patient needs treatment in this case, and the prognosis is perhaps not as good. Then ask questions that will raise concerns that this patient might have a more serious cause of their pain. These include weight loss, anorexia, fever, dysphagia, odynophagia, and hoarse voice, all of which mandate careful neck examination for masses, adenopathy, and oropharyngeal lesions. X-rays, bone scan and/or CT scan would then be pursued.

Otherwise, the history of when the pain is present, and what positions aggravate it are less useful, except to determine that the pain is worse with activity or at the end of the day. This affirms a suspicion that the patient has a benign cause for their pain.

Examination of the cervical spine

Normal ranges of motion are:

Flexion	45°
Extension	60°
Lateral rotation	80°
Lateral flexion	45°

The examination proceeds as follows:

1. Ask the patient to locate their pain. The larger the area of pain, the more likely they have a chronic pain syndrome.

2. Ask the patient to touch their chin to their chest, then their ears towards their shoulders, then look up at the ceiling, and look to the right and left. This range will be normal with patients with mechanical neck pain or chronic pain syndromes, with pain at the extremes of the range.

   If their range is limited, have them relax as you gently achieve passive range of motion. If this is abnormal (limited in a patient who is relaxed), then examine the remainder of the spine, specifically looking for ankylosing spondylitis (see the section on seronegative spondylo-arthropathy, page 133.)

3. Pressing over the posterior aspect of the cervical spine to find some tender spot is not very useful. If just light pressure causes pain over just one of the vertebrae, however, then the patient is either malingering, has an exaggerated pain response (chronic pain syndrome), or has a serious problem. To test for the first two, use some of the tips from the section above on the painful back). If they do not confirm your suspicions, then X-rays, and bone scan at least are needed.

4. Finally, check the reflexes and muscle strength of the arms. Testing for sensation is not as useful, as frequently patients with chronic pain syndromes will describe poor sensation in their arms which does not conform to a dermatomal distribution.

As for investigations, it should be realized that just as for the lumbar spine, there is a poor correlation between X-ray findings and neck pain. Pain may be severe with normal X-rays, and markedly abnormal neck X-rays may be found in an asymptomatic individual. More importantly, the majority of people over 50 will have abnormalities. Even 5% of the general population under 40 years of age may have abnormalities. It is equally true that up to 30% of the young, asymptomatic population may have abnormalities on CT scan or MRI. If an MRI is ordered on a patient with fibromyalgia, you might find disc protrusion, and be tempted to refer the patient for surgery. You may be ascribing their symptoms to a finding that is not clinically relevant. You should only therefore be ordering such tests for specific reasons (i.e. the patient has an absent biceps reflex on the left side and muscle weakness in elbow flexion) and you are looking for the disc protrusion on the left side at the C5–C6 level, and may refer to a surgeon. Spinal stenosis can also be an incidental finding, and unless neurological signs can be attributed to this stenosis, it is not of consequence (i.e. pain alone is not an indication for doing anything about spinal stenosis, particularly when there is no objective clinical evidence that the stenosis is relevant.)

Management

The management of neck pain due to a chronic pain syndrome is as for that described in the sections on these illnesses. Similarly, for mechanical neck pain exercises are recommended (see Appendix 6), emphasizing that the patient does not have to worry that this problem will disable or paralyze them, or cause crippling arthritis of the neck.

Although some believe neck traction to be of benefit, some do not. There are as many ways to treat neck pain as there are for back pain, but the key is to not give the patient a dismal prognosis, but rather let them know that this is not a crippling disease.

While neck collars are often used, they may be harmful. If they are worn day and night, the patient will find they have pain as soon as they remove them. Insisting that they wear them only during the day, or only when they have most of their pain, or not using them at all are better alternatives to dependency on them.

Patients with whiplash complain of neck pain, of course, and some believe that these patients have a chronic pain syndrome, and should be treated with recommendations given previously for those illnesses.

Finally, see also the section on rheumatoid arthritis (page 117) for the assessment and management of neck pain in this condition.

DOs and DON'Ts of Neck Pain

DO ask about weight loss, fever, bladder or bowel incontinence, and nocturnal onset of neck pain. Some of these patients will have diseases other than mechanical neck pain.

DO remember that patients with chronic pain syndromes present with neck pain.

DO explain to the patient that readiness to return to work is not determined by lack of pain. They will have pain when they return to work, but will not damage their neck from doing so.

DO recommend neck exercises.

DON'T tell the patient they will have a progressive arthritis of the spine. They will not, but if enough people tell them so a chronic pain syndrome will develop.

DON'T routinely order X-rays. Explain to the patient that X-rays are not needed at this time, but will be considered only if symptoms persist or worsen despite the patient's attempts at appropriate exercises.

DON'T order CT or MRI scans unless one has clear, objective clinical findings suggestive of disc protrusion with neurologic deficit. Pain is not an indication for these scans, no matter how severe.

DON'T let patients become obsessed with X-ray findings.

DON'T treat chronic neck pain with narcotics.

DON'T prescribe dependency on collars for neck pain.

DON'T allow the patient to become dependent on regular physiotherapy visits, but instead encourage independent home therapy.

Section 5 – Outside the algorithm

> # Systemic sclerosis

When a patient complains of distal finger pain and tightening, or develops pits on their fingertips, or has true Raynaud's phenomenon, consider scleroderma.

Systemic sclerosis is a multisystem disease characterized by inflammatory, vascular, and fibrotic changes of the skin and visceral organs. Strictly speaking, the term 'scleroderma' refers to the skin disease alone, but it is often used in place of systemic sclerosis, since there are only a few rare conditions which may otherwise produce this skin disease. It affects mostly women between 30 and 50 years of age, but children and the elderly can be affected. The disease is not always progressive and may reverse. Visceral organ involvement may precede the skin manifestations, and the disease may be rapidly progressive or indolent.

Table 5.1 Clinical manifestations of systemic sclerosis

Skin
    Scleroderma
    Telangiectasias
    Skin breakdown over bony prominences
    Calcinosis
Joints
    Arthralgias/arthritis
    Contractures
Cardiovascular
    Raynaud's phenomenon
    Pericarditis
    Congestive heart failure
    Conduction defects
    Supraventricular or ventricular dysrhythmias
Pulmonary
    Interstitial fibrosis
    Pulmonary hypertension
    Lung cancer
Renal
    Scleroderma crisis
Gastrointestinal
    Dysphagia
    Hypomobility
    Malabsorption
Miscellaneous
    Sjögren's syndrome
    Hypothyroidism

It is thought to be due to overproduction of normal collagen, the primary event perhaps being endothelial injury of small arteries or capillaries, with eventual fibrosis occurring in affected tissues. The tissues are edematous initially due to the inflammation, then the edema resolves as collagen deposition is taking place. The final phase is consolidation and contraction of the fibrosis. Vascular obliteration leads to dilation of other capillaries (telangiectasias).

Systemic sclerosis can have either diffuse scleroderma (rapidly progressing, widespread skin disease including trunk, and early visceral involvement) or limited scleroderma (distal limbs and face, with late visceral involvement). The latter is closely related to the CREST syndrome (Calcinosis, Raynaud's phenomenon, Esophageal hypomotility, Sclerodactyly, and Telangiectasias). See *Table 5.1* for the disease manifestations, with a discussion of some important ones below.

Clinical manifestations and treatment

Raynaud's phenomenon (90% of patients with skin disease) sometimes precedes other manifestations by years. It is treated as described previously for SLE. The fingers and hands become swollen, then gradually become leathery. These changes may involve chiefly the distal limbs (limited scleroderma) or include the trunk (diffuse scleroderma). The soft pulp of the fingertips can be lost and ulcers may appear there as well over bony prominences if the skin is too tight. Skin may be hyper- or hypopigmented, and telangiectasias may appear (also seen in nail beds). Normal facial wrinkles are lost and the mouth may be difficult to open. There have been many proposed therapies for the skin disease, most commonly penicillamine starting at 250 mg qd increasing by 250 mg every 2 months to a tolerated dose of 750–1000 mg qd. Other therapies tried include colchicine, azathioprine, methotrexate, cyclosporin, cyclophosphamide, photopheresis, interferons, and retinoids. There are no controlled trials to prove their efficacy.

Dry skin should be treated with emollients. Skin ulcers may be treated with occlusive dressings and local debridement. If they appear infected, and deep infection is ruled out, oral antibiotics may be used, otherwise intravenous antibiotics and more extensive surgical measures may be needed. Patients are encouraged to exercise joint range of motion and orofacial motion. If joint contractures or deformities are severe, joint fusion is sometimes used to improve hand function.

Patients may have symmetric polyarthritis (50%) that can be treated with NSAIDs and carpal tunnel syndrome (tendon thickening). Patients may develop a myopathy. Sometimes this myopathy appears on biopsy to be like polymyositis (and responds to corticosteroids), but there is also a form which does not appear to be the same as polymyositis and does not respond to corticosteroids. Calcinosis is difficult to treat, although colchicine may be helpful.

There is no good therapy for pulmonary hypertension. Pericarditis is treated with NSAIDs or prednisone (prednisolone), while dysrhythmias and heart failure are treated in standard ways. Pulmonary fibrosis may possibly respond to penicillamine, or other immunosuppressives, especially cyclophosphamide. Lung cancer is a late complication of the disease.

Renal involvement may begin in the first 2 years and renal failure can rapidly occur. Proteinuria, abnormal sediment, hypertension, azotemia, and micro-angiopathic hemolytic anemia are features associated with progressive renal disease. In particular, a 'renal crisis' may occur and is characterized by accelerated or malignant hypertension and rapidly declining renal function. There is substantial evidence that the outcome of scleroderma renal crisis can be modified by the early and aggressive use of angiotensin-converting enzyme inhibitors, but general measures for treatment of malignant hypertension are also important (admission to monitored bed, arterial pressure monitoring, and sometimes concomitant use of other vasodilators). It is important to regularly monitor all scleroderma patients for hypertension, and treat it aggressively. Corticosteroids should be avoided in scleroderma as they have been shown to increase the risk of a renal crisis.

Esophageal involvement (50%) may lead to heartburn, strictures, dysphagia, and delayed gastric emptying. Small intestine involvement may lead to bloating, abdominal pain, ileus, constipation (large intestine), and small bowel diverticulae.

Reflux symptoms may improve with anti-reflux measures (inclined bed, small, frequent meals), H_2-blockers, or omeprazole (20 mg qd) and cisapride (10 mg qid) or metoclopramide (10 mg qid). Esophageal strictures may be dilated, and surgical procedures to improve lower esophageal sphincter dysfunction may be successful. Malabsorption (particularly with steatorrhea) is often due to bacterial overgrowth and should be given a trial of antibiotics (like metronidazole for a few weeks).

A summary of drug therapy of systemic sclerosis is given in *Table 5.2*.

Table 5.2 Summary of drug therapy of systemic sclerosis

Manifestation	Therapy
Scleroderma	Penicillamine, colchicine, or other immuno suppressives
Skin ulcers	Occlusive dressings, antibiotics if infected
Calcinosis	None proven
Sjögren's syndrome	Artificial tears, frequent fluid intake
Arthritis	NSAIDs
Pericarditis	NSAIDs or corticosteroids
Esophageal involvement	H_2-blockers or omeprazole
Esophageal or bowel dysmotility	Metoclopramide or cisapride
Malabsorption	Consider antibiotics
Raynaud's phenomenon	Nifedipine, prazosin, or captopril

Laboratory findings

ANA, anti-Scl-70 antibodies, anti-RNP antibodies, (including anti-nucleolar antibodies) rheumatoid factor, and hypergammaglobulinemia may be found. The CREST syndrome typically has anti-centromere antibodies alone. Hand X-rays may show terminal phalangeal bone resorption and calcinosis.

DOs and DON'Ts of Systemic Sclerosis (Scleroderma)

DO have the patient seen by a rheumatologist, and gastroenterologist if GI involvement.

DON'T use corticosteroids unless recommended by a rheumatologist.

DON'T overdiagnose Raynaud's phenomenon in patients who really do not have this condition.

Section 5 – Outside the algorithm

Polymyositis and dermatomyositis

When a patient complains of weakness in the limbs (with pain a lesser symptom), one must consider a neuropathy or myopathy. In myositis, the patient will complain of leg weakness (getting out of a chair, climbing stairs), and arm weakness (reaching above their head, combing their hair).

Polymyositis and dermatomyositis are diseases of unknown cause, characterized chiefly by proximal muscle weakness, and in the case of dermatomyositis, a specific rash. Both children and adults may be affected, adult women being the most common. There is an association of these diseases with malignancy in adults (not children), especially dermatomyositis. Mostly striated muscle is involved, but cardiac and smooth muscle may also be involved. Myositis must be distinguished from fibromyalgia and polymyalgia rheumatica (CK levels and ESR are helpful: see sections on chronic pain syndromes (page 26) and polymyalgia rheumatica (page 39)).

Clinical manifestations and treatment

These are listed in *Table 5.3* and some are discussed below.

Patients experience a symmetric, occasionally painful, proximal muscle weakness of the limbs and trunk, producing difficulty in climbing stairs, arising from a sitting position, and raising the arms above the shoulders. There may be oropharyngeal dysphagia and nasal phonation (palatal weakness) in advanced cases. Very few progress to involve distal muscles. The patient may have malaise, fatigue, and weight loss as well.

To look for proximal muscle weakness, ask the patient to lift their head off the examining table when downward pressure is placed on the forehead, to hold their arms out at 90° and resist downward pressure, to flex their hips against resistance, and to squat and then stand. Normal muscles can perform these tasks quite well. With individuals who have a well developed musculature (particularly young men), myositis may exist with no evidence of weakness with the above tests. They should be tested by doing push-ups, or repeated squatting. A normal young man should be able to squat 10 times easily, or do 10 push-ups.

Table 5.3   Clinical manifestations of polymyositis and dermatomyositis

Skin
    Heliotrope rash
    Gottron's papules
    Red-purple rash
    Nail capillary telangiectasias
    Vasculitis
    Calcinosis

Pulmonary
    Ventilatory (muscle) failure
    Aspiration pneumonia
    Hypersensitivity pneumonitis
    Opportunistic infections
    Interstitial lung disease
    Pulmonary hypertension (rare)
    Pulmonary vasculitis (rare)

Cardiac
    Heart block
    Dysrhythmias
    Cardiomyopathy

Gastrointestinal
    Oropharyngeal dysphagia
    Lower esophageal dysphagia
    Intestinal hypomotility

Musculoskeletal
    Proximal muscle weakness
    Distal muscle weakness (uncommon)
    Arthritis

Once the diagnosis is confirmed by muscle biopsy, start prednisone (prednisolone) at 60–80 mg qd for about 6–8 weeks. If the patient is significantly improved and the CK level is returning to normal, the dosage can be gradually reduced by 5–10 mg every month to usually a maintenance of 5–10 mg qd (or 10–20 mg alternate days). The most important marker of disease activity and therapy efficacy is symptoms and quantitative muscle strength. A crude measure is grading strength as 0–5. (0 is no purposeful muscle movement at all, 1 is trace movement, 2 is movement only when not against gravity, 3 is able to resist gravity, 4 is able to resist gravity and additional force from an examiner, and 5 is normal.) Others use formal myometry, and the time it takes for the patient to stand 10 times from sitting, without using the hands.

If the patient's symptoms recur or worsen, then an increase in the dosage to the previous effective level is required. Some patients may have slight, persistent elevations in CK levels with no change in symptoms. They can be observed at a stable dose if they are clinically stable. Further elevations in the CK level often herald a clinical worsening, but it is preferable that changes in therapy be guided by the changes in clinical findings, not solely the CK level.

Failure to respond to corticosteroids after 12 weeks, inability to taper corticosteroids, failure to respond fully, and inability to tolerate corticosteroids are indications for other therapy. One must be confident of the diagnosis, however. Methotrexate may be added 15 mg/week orally, subcutaneously, intravenously or intramuscularly (rarely causes an elevated CK level), increasing every few weeks by 10 mg/week up to 50 mg/week if needed (although this may not be well tolerated). When muscle strength starts to improve and the CK level is also improving (does not have to be normal, but close), the corticosteroids can be tapered off completely. At doses over 20 mg, oral methotrexate may not be well tolerated or absorbed, so a parenteral route is often needed. An alternative to methotrexate includes azathioprine 100–150 mg qd until the patient can be tapered off corticosteroids, then azathioprine 50–75 mg qd for maintenance. Chlorambucil, cyclophosphamide, cyclosporin, and IV immunoglobulin are other therapies that have been tried in refractory cases.

Patients who have been on prolonged corticosteroids (especially high dose > 1 year) may have worsening symptoms due to corticosteroid myopathy. Repeat muscle biopsy and EMG studies may be helpful to determine the disease activity in these cases. Otherwise a patient with corticosteroid myopathy may incorrectly be given more corticosteroids.

Physiotherapy and occupational therapy are useful. They help to improve function and coping during the periods of muscle weakness, and also to maintain muscle flexibility, since patients may otherwise develop flexion contractures.

The rash of dermatomyositis occurs chiefly on the face, chest, and extensor surfaces of the extremities. It is red-purple, slightly raised and finely scaling. When it appears periorbital it is referred to as heliotrope rash, and over the knuckles it is referred to as Gottron's papules. The rash may respond to antimalarials as well as other disease therapies. Cutaneous vasculitis in dermatomyositis manifests as tender nodules and digital ulcerations. Corticosteroid therapy is effective for the vasculitis.

Calcinosis occurs in the muscle fascia and subcutaneous tissues as a late manifestation, and is more of a problem in pediatric cases. The involved areas may form large areas that become inflamed and open to the surface draining the material. This is difficult to treat, although drugs like colchicine and etidronate have been tried. It may be prevented by adequate disease therapy in the first place.

Ventilation is impaired by respiratory muscle weakness. In addition, 15% of patients may develop pulmonary fibrosis with dyspnea, cough, and hypoxemia. This often requires agents such as cyclophosphamide for therapy, but the prognosis is poor. Aspiration pneumonia may occur, and therefore new onset of pulmonary infiltrates should prompt a search for infection. As well, at high doses, methotrexate may induce a hypersensitivity pneumonitis, requiring its withdrawal. (It is not usually used in patients with pre-existing lung disease.)

At the time of diagnosis there is an association between the presence of malignancy and myositis. Those with established disease, however, do not appear to be at any greater risk of developing malignancy in the future. Most malignancies will be found by history and physical examination (including breast and pelvic examination), stool examination for occult blood, CBC, urinalysis, mammography, pelvic and vaginal ultrasound (women), and chest X-ray. Older patients are more likely to have a malignancy. The myositis may improve with tumor excision.

Laboratory findings

The diagnosis is based on the clinical findings, electromyography, and muscle biopsy. The CK level may be normal early in the disease, but a repeat

Table 5.4 Differential diagnosis of polymyositis/dermatomyositis

Metabolic/Endocrine
  Hypo/hyperthyroidism
  Cushing's syndrome
  Hypocalcemia
  Hypokalemia
  Diabetic amyotrophy/neuropathy

Drugs
  Alcohol
  Corticosteroids
  Colchicine
  Zidovudine (AZT)
  Lovastatin
  D-penicillamine
  Chloroquine

Myopathies
  Limb-girdle dystrophy
  Fascioscapulohumeral dystrophy
  Congenital muscular dystrophies
  Myotonic dystrophy

Neuromuscular
  Motor neuron disease (poliomyelitis, amyotrophic lateral sclerosis)
  Myasthenia gravis
  Idiopathic radicular polyneuritis (e.g. Guillain-Barre syndrome)

Infections
  Viral (HIV, coxsackie, influenza, Epstein-Barr, cytomegalovirus)
  Bacterial (Lyme disease, mycoplasma, leprosy, tuberculosis)
  Fungal (candida)
  Parasitic (trichinosis, cysticercosis, trypanosomiasis)

Other rheumatic diseases
  Polymyalgia rheumatica
  Fibrositis
  Scleroderma
  SLE
  Sjögren's syndrome
  Rheumatoid arthritis

determination in a few weeks will likely show elevation. A biopsy-proven diagnosis is preferred in all cases. The biopsy should be done by an experienced individual and in co-operation with an experienced pathologist. The deltoid or quadriceps muscles are most commonly used. The same muscle should not be used for EMG and biopsy. The muscle to be biopsied should not have had a recent (1 week) intra-muscular injection.

A differential diagnosis of other common causes of myositis is presented in *Table 5.4*. One should always check the patient's drug list and the appropriate drug reference book, as many medications may cause an elevated CK level or myositis. Muscle biopsy effectively separates these from polymyositis. It is rare to have extra-ocular muscles involved, so this would prompt one to consider myasthenia gravis or multiple sclerosis.

Serology may reveal one of a number of different autoantibodies which are myositis-specific. These are not required for diagnosis, but include anti-Jo-1 antibodies which identify individuals at higher risk for pulmonary fibrosis. The ESR and creatine kinase are elevated. In polymyalgia rheumatica the ESR is elevated and CK level is normal. In fibromyalgia both the ESR and CK level should be normal. As well, pain is prominent in polymyalgia rheumatica and fibromyalgia, and nonexistent or mild in polymyositis.

There are occasional patients with myositis who do not have elevated CK levels. If a patient has objective proximal muscle weakness, and a normal CK level, referral to a rheumatologist, and muscle biopsy are worthwhile.

DOs and DON'Ts of Myositis

DO have a rheumatologist confirm the diagnosis, or obtain a muscle biopsy/EMG to prove the diagnosis.

DO remember to adequately stress a muscular individual before concluding there is no muscle weakness.

DO confirm that the CK level returns to normal (or near normal) with therapy.

DO refer to a rheumatologist if unable to taper corticosteroids to less than 20 mg in a few months due to recurrence of symptoms.

DO continue to taper corticosteroids even if the CK level is mildly abnormal, as long as the patient is asymptomatic.

DON'T use the CK level alone to guide therapy.

Section 5 – Outside the algorithm

Vasculitis

Whenever confronted with a patient who has unexplained systemic symptomatology (fever, weight loss, night sweats), palpable purpura, mononeuritis multiplex, or organ failure, the vasculitides should be considered.

Patients with these symptoms are often investigated for malignancy, and chronic infection. Pursuing the diagnosis of vasculitis if these are negative is worthwhile. One does not actually need to know a great deal about the various forms of vasculitis to make a diagnosis. It is much simpler than that: find a tissue site to biopsy. When that site is found, refer to the appropriate specialist with the concern of looking for vasculitis and wait for the pathologist to send back a diagnosis.

Table 5.5   In search of vasculitis

Symptom or sign	Investigation and referral
Temporal or occipital headache Visual loss Jaw claudication Tender temporal arteries	ESR and temporal artery biopsy
Stroke syndrome (especially in young patient)	CT or MRI scan and neurologist
Seizure disorder in adult age > 20	CT or MRI scan and neurologist
Eye lesions or inflammation	Ophthalmologist
Nosebleeds or nasal septum ulceration Hoarse voice	Ear nose and throat surgeon

Cough, hemoptysis, dyspnea, recurrent
  sinusitis
	Chest X-ray and other scans,
	  pulmonologist (Chest physician)

Gastrointestinal bleeds (especially lower)	Endoscopy and gastroenterologist
Bowel perforation	Surgical biopsy
Proteinuria Hematuria Cellular casts in urine	Nephrologist
Unexplained skin rash, nodule, or ulcer	Dermatologist
Weakness or sensory loss in a specific peripheral nerve (mononeuritis multiplex)	Neurologist

When looking for a tissue biopsy site (which will determine what investigations and referrals are needed), take clues from the history and examination. Proceed from the head down (*Table 5.5*).

The patient complaining of episodic numbness or weakness in the hand or foot does not have a mononeuritis multiplex. Instead they should describe, for example, persistent numbness of medial forearm and 4th and 5th digits with weakness of these digits (ulnar nerve) or foot drop (peroneal nerve). There should be objective findings. Do not chase after intermittent and nonspecific paresthesias as being vasculitis. When nerve involvement occurs, it produces very obvious symptoms and signs.

If you cannot find a site of involvement by history, examination, or these investigations, it is highly unlikely that a vasculitis exists.

One simplified method of classification divides the vasculitides by the size of the vessels involved (i.e. capillaries, arterioles, or venules; small or medium-sized arteries; and large arteries). Since these different sized vessels appear in or near most organs, all forms of vasculitis can involve each of these organs. Vasculitis may be a primary disease or associated with other rheumatic diseases, infection, drugs, and malignancy. A classification scheme is presented in *Table 5.6*. The more common forms of vasculitis will be discussed.

Table 5.6 Classification of vasculitis

Capillaries, arterioles, or venules
      Henoch-Schonlein purpura
      Hypersensitivity vasculitis
      Rheumatoid arthritis
      SLE
      Sjögren's syndrome
      Polymyositis
      Cryoglobulinemia
      Subacute bacterial endocarditis
      Chronic active hepatitis
      Inflammatory bowel disease
      Malignancy (mostly hematologic)
      Behcet's disease

Small and medium-sized arteries
      Polyarteritis nodosa (classic or microscopic)
      Wegener's granulomatosis
      Rheumatoid arthritis (rare)
      Behcet's disease

Large arteries
      Giant cell (temporal) arteritis
      Takayasu's arteritis
      Behcet's disease

Small-vessel (capillary, arteriole, or venule) vasculitis

This form of vasculitis is referred to by many terms, including hypersensitivity vasculitis, hypersensitivity venulitis, Henoch-Schonlein purpura, post-capillary angiitis, leucocytoclastic vasculitis, and allergic vasculitis. As a group, they account for more than 90% of vasculitides. Cutaneous manifestations dominate, and serious organ dysfunction is uncommon. Many cases are idiopathic, but common causes include drugs, infections (e.g. Hepatitis B, bacteria), and foreign proteins.

Skin involvement occurs chiefly over the lower limbs, buttocks, and trunk with lesions that include palpable purpura (non-blanching lesions), macules, vesicles, hemorrhagic bullae, and ulcers. Patients often have fever, malaise, gastrointestinal symptoms (abdominal pain, nausea, diarrhea, bleeding), and arthralgias/arthritis. Other organ involvement is much less common, but renal, neurologic, and pulmonary disease can occur.

Henoch-Schonlein purpura is a typical idiopathic form of this vasculitis, more common in children, but also seen in adults. The rash (palpable purpura) typically occurs over the lower limbs, but may be more widespread. Patients often develop abdominal pain, arthralgias or arthritis, and much less commonly gastrointestinal bleeding. Proteinuria and red cell casts are seen. Most cases remit spontaneously in 1–2 weeks, so that often patients are treated symptomatically with NSAIDs, for example. Corticosteroids (prednisone (prednisolone) 1 mg/kg/d) may be given for prolonged or unresponsive cases, tapering over a few weeks. Unresolving proteinuria or renal cell casts warrant further assessment by a nephrologist.

Other systemic rheumatic diseases, cryoglobulinemia, subacute bacterial endocarditis, hematologic malignancies, and drugs may cause small-vessel vasculitis.

Small and medium-sized artery vasculitis

Polyarteritis nodosa
Polyarteritis nodosa is a serious systemic necrotizing vasculitis (necrosis is in vessel wall). It produces organ failure, as do many other forms of vasculitis, by the ultimate mechanism of ischemic infarction. There is an association between hepatitis B antigenemia and polyarteritis nodosa. Microscopic polyarteritis nodosa is a related disease which may have similar disease involvement and therapy.

Fever, malaise, headache, myalgias, arthralgias, weight loss, and hypertension are common.

The cutaneous involvement produces painful, erythematous, subcutaneous nodules, or may produce livedo reticularis.

Renal involvement includes hypertension, frank ischemia, glomerulonephritis, or nephrosclerosis with possible findings of proteinuria, hematuria, and/or red cell casts.

Gastrointestinal involvement ranges from mild nausea and abdominal pain to infarction of bowel or other intra-abdominal viscus, and perforation. Liver disease may be due to infarction or be a complication of hepatitis B infection.

Coronary artery involvement may lead to infarction, otherwise pericarditis and congestive heart failure may occur. Pulmonary involvement is rarely seen.

Mononeuritis multiplex, cutaneous neuropathy, polyneuropathy, and cerebro-vascular involvement also occurs.

Unusual sites of involvement may produce epididymitis and testicular pain. Muscle involvement may be very painful.

The diagnosis generally requires tissue biopsy, directed initially at the involved organ, although blind rectal muscle, or testicular biopsy can sometimes be positive. It has been suggested that the characteristic angiographic findings in bowel and renal vessel involvement (multiple aneurysms) in the appropriate clinical setting are sufficient for diagnosis and treatment, if no other site of involvement can be found.

It is important to look for hepatitis B antigenemia (although rare in the UK), since the liver disease may have its own morbidity, and sometimes requires specific anti-viral therapy.

Therapy depends on the severity of disease involvement. It is not necessary to treat cutaneous disease unless severe. Colchicine alone has been effective in some cases. More severe cutaneous disease may be treated with high-dose corticosteroids, for example prednisone (prednisolone) 1 mg/kg/d for 4 weeks, then 0.5 mg/kg for 4 weeks, and continue tapering over several months, assuming the patient continues to do well.

More significant organ involvement (renal, neurologic, cardiac, gastrointestinal) warrants combined therapy with corticosteroids and cyclophosphamide. Imminent organ failure definitely requires combination therapy. Other indications for cyclophosphamide include failure to improve after 1 month of corticosteroids. Cyclophosphamide without corticosteroids is not used, since it often takes 2–3 weeks for its full benefit to be apparent. Cyclophosphamide may be given as oral 2 mg/kg/d. Most American rheumatologists recommend oral cyclophosphamide over intravenous form, especially for severe forms of vasculitis. (Nevertheless, there are a number of Canadian and British rheumatologists who use either intravenous cyclophosphamide alone, or intravenous followed eventually by oral therapy. Intravenously, it is given as 15 mg/kg (maximum 1000 mg) every 2 weeks initially, then every 3 weeks). There is considerable variability in the duration of therapy chosen, but 1–2 years is commonly used.

Oral cyclophosphamide may be more often associated with hemorrhagic cystitis which produces pain and microscopic or gross hematuria, and is diagnosed by cystoscopy. Its occurrence means therapy must be held until the hematuria completely resolves, but it may be restarted if the episode was mild. Some routinely use oral mesna to prevent this toxicity. Malignancy with oral cyclophosphamide is unfortunately a complication in up to 5% of cases (bladder cancer), and 1% will develop hematologic malignancies. Any patient on cyclophosphamide requires urinalysis (looking for hematuria) every 6 months. There are some who recommend lifetime surveillance. Other adverse effects include pancytopenia, gonadal dysfunction (especially ovarian), and pulmonary or bladder fibrosis. Thus, one must judge the severity of the vasculitis before accepting these risks.

Cyclophosphamide dose must be decreased in renal failure (< 5–10 mg/kg IV, < 0.5–1.0 mg/kg oral). All patients should have monthly or pre-pulse CBC and renal function tests.

Azathioprine, methotrexate, pulse high-dose IV corticosteroids, plasmapheresis, and chlorambucil have been used in some cases.

Relapse after remission is infrequent.

Wegener's granulomatosis

Wegener's granulomatosis is also a systemic, serious necrotizing vasculitis, but has a different clinicopathologic appearance than polyarteritis nodosa. Many of the symptoms described above occur, but there is a predilection for involvement of the upper and lower respiratory tract (including sinuses, nose, ears, larynx), and kidneys. The pulmonary involvement is a key distinguishing clinical feature from polyarteritis nodosa.

Symptoms and signs include rhinorrhea, sinusitis, nasal mucosal ulcerations, epistaxis, cough, hemoptysis, otitis, dyspnea, scleritis, episcleritis, and iritis. Inflammatory nodules may appear on the ear pinna. Chest X-ray may reveal a bilateral reticulonodular pattern, or multiple nodules with or without cavitation. Pleural effusions and atelectasis may be seen, but adenopathy is usually not seen.

Renal disease is in the form of focal or diffuse glomerulonephritis, and can be rapidly progressive. A skin rash or scleral nodule may also be a complication seen.

Secondary infection with *S. aureus* may occur in the respiratory tract when involved. This may be confused with a recurrence or worsening of the disease, and it is of course important to rule infection out or treat it if present, because intensifying immunosuppressive therapy may be detrimental in this case.

Anti-neutrophil cytoplasmic antibodies (ANCA) are often found, but the diagnosis should still be made by biopsy where possible. The differential diagnosis of pulmonary involvement is, of course, large, but many of these conditions can be diagnosed by lung biopsy. It is reasonable to start with bronchoscopy, but if inconclusive results are obtained, an open lung biopsy is indicated.

Both corticosteroids and cyclophosphamide are used as described for polyarteritis nodosa, but recurrences are more common with Wegener's granulomatosis. There is an emerging body of literature suggesting that methotrexate may be an alternative to cyclophosphamide. Nevertheless, cyclophosphamide should be used in combination with prednisone (prednisolone) in all patients presenting with renal involvement and may be necessary in those with severe respiratory involvement.

Medium and large-sized artery vasculitis

Giant cell arteritis (temporal arteritis)
Whenever an elderly patient presents with new onset headache (usually temporal or occipital), an episode of visual loss, diplopia, or jaw pain, check the ESR.

Giant cell arteritis typically affects a much older age group than the other vasculitides (it is rare before the age of 50 years). It can affect any branch of the aorta, but most commonly the external or internal carotid arteries (also called cranial arteritis). The classic one is giant cell arteritis with fever, anemia, myalgias, visual disturbance, and an elevated ESR. There may be any of headache, jaw claudication, visual loss, blurring, or diplopia.

There is an association with polymyalgia rheumatica (stiffness and myalgias in shoulders, upper back, neck, hips, and thighs), occuring in 40% of patients, and about 20% of patients with polymyalgia rheumatica may have symptoms of arteritis. Mild synovitis of large joints has been described. Patients may have symptoms or signs of vascular compromise elsewhere, such as limb ischemia, Raynaud's phenomenon, jaw claudication, and tongue claudication. The temporal arteries may, but do not have to, be tender.

The ESR is usually markedly elevated (> 80 for Westergren), but there have been cases diagnosed in the presence of a normal ESR, these patients having otherwise typical symptoms and a positive biopsy. The CK level will be normal. The diagnosis should be supported by biopsy. The biopsy most likely to be positive is that in which the temporal artery sample is over 2 cm in length. The opposite artery may have to be biopsied if the first is negative, and the clinical suspicion still exists. If the diagnosis is strongly suspected clinically (symptoms and high ESR), but the biopsy is negative, begin therapy and refer to a rheumatologist for further advice.

Give prednisone (prednisolone) 40–60 mg qd, to 30 mg qd in the second month (if symptoms have remitted) and then gradually taper over several months, to a maintenance dose of 5 mg qd or alternate days. The usual duration of therapy is for at least 1–2 years. The dose is tapered according to the patient's symptoms. Recurrence of symptoms warrants a return to a dosage usually of 20–30 mg qd. One should not rely on the ESR alone to guide dosage adjustments since it may remain mildly abnormal despite effective treatment, or it may be normal despite symptoms.

Therapy should be started immediately, particularly in the setting of visual disturbance, jaw claudication, or pulse abnormalities since a delay while waiting too long for biopsy may lead to blindness. Instead, one should initiate therapy, and obtain the biopsy within 2–3 days so as not to alter the diagnostic yield (waiting more than 1 week may give false-negative biopsy results). Note that polymyalgia rheumatica alone is also treated with corticosteroids, but at a much lower dose. (See the topic on polymyalgia rheumatica, page 39).

DOs and DON'Ts of Vasculitis

DO consider vasculitis in a patient with unexplained systemic symptoms (weight loss, fever, night sweats) and look for something to biopsy to confirm vasculitis.

DO order an ESR on elderly patients who present with headache, visual loss, diplopia, or jaw pain.

DO confirm clinical diagnosis of giant cell arteritis by biopsy, and do not delay therapy while waiting for biopsy (but get a biopsy within a few days). If the biopsy is negative, but one still suspects the diagnosis, consult a rheumatologist, while continuing therapy.

DO consult a rheumatologist if the biopsy is positive for vasculitis.

DO involve a rheumatologist whenever corticosteroid therapy is being considered. The tapering, and adjustment of corticosteroid dosage, especially in giant cell arteritis, can be difficult in some patients. Given that they are expected to be on long term corticosteroids, it is worthwhile to have a rheumatologist help with these decisions.

DON'T order serology as a screen. It is useful only in very specific settings.

DON'T increase corticosteroid dose for nonspecific symptoms like malaise, fatigue, nausea, or generalized aches. If unsure of whether or not to increase the dose, or if a patient seems to complain of these symptoms every time the dose is lowered, consult a rheumatologist.

Reflex sympathetic dystrophy

When a patient presents with a diffuse pain in the upper or lower limb, and that limb was seen by a physician to be diffusely swollen, consider reflex sympathetic dystrophy. Arthritis does not produce this type of swelling. Obviously, if the hand has been swollen for 4 weeks, it is not cellulitis or trauma. If the symptoms have been present only for a few days or a week, one may have to consider cellulitis or deep venous thrombosis (in the leg), but after this period reflex sympathetic dystrophy is virtually the only possibility. It is often very painful, and the skin is sensitive to touch. One might confuse this with regional myofascial pain syndrome, but remember that chronic pain syndromes do not produce objective swelling. (Remember that any time a patient complains of swelling, it must be objectively documented by a physician.)

This label is sometimes given to patients who actually have a chronic pain syndrome, usually because the patient complained of swelling, but no one verified that swelling actually occurred.

Reflex sympathetic dystrophy often follows a specific triggering event. The regions most commonly involved are the entire upper limb, hand, shoulder, single digits, entire lower limb, hip, knee, foot, and patella. It may follow trauma (may be minor), surgical procedures, burns, frostbite, strokes, peripheral neuropathy (like spinal nerve impingement), prolonged immobilization, pregnancy, or barbiturate use.

The first phase (1–6 months) is pain and swelling weeks or months after the event, burning pain and warmth, increased sweating and hair growth. In the second phase, the skin becomes thin, shiny, and cool. In the third phase, Dupuytren's contracture may occur and the limb becomes significantly restricted in motion. Physical examination shows marked tenderness, and edema (may be pitting), and restriction of motion (that is usually improved on passive movement). There may be erythema or pallor, decreased hair growth, brittle nails, and increased sweating. In late phases, skin and subcutaneous atrophy may occur.

Radiographs may show mottled osteopenia of the affected region early, then more diffuse osteopenia. The bone scan will show increased activity diffusely in the affected region, and in late stages, in the bone. **If one has not witnessed** the swelling the patient claims to have had, and therefore one is not sure the patient does not simply have a chronic pain syndrome, radiographs will help diagnose reflex sympathetic dystrophy. The diagnosis is made largely on the basis of clinical findings, with these radiologic changes (which may not always be present, however). Sympathetic blocks are sometimes diagnostic if they relieve symptoms. The key is, however, to have clearly documented swelling.

The patient should be reassured that they do not have arthritis. They must be strongly encouraged to stretch fully and exercise the limb daily. NSAIDs may provide some analgesia to make such exercises easier, but the patient must know that although they may experience more pain with these exercises, they are not doing harm, and it is exercise, not medication, that is the mainstay of therapy. The exercises which can be used are included in Appendices 2, 3 and 4, depending on which limb is affected. Occasionally, regional sympathetic blocks with quanethidine, for example, are used and may be the most effective form of therapy. These measures alone are effective in mild cases. In moderate or severe cases, prednisone (prednisolone) 60–80 mg qd tapered over 1 month (when swelling is present) or calcitonin 50 µg subcutaneous bid for a few weeks may be helpful early in the disease (may be tried at any stage, however). In late disease, medical therapy may not be effective, but persistent physiotherapy must be maintained if recovery is to occur (which may take months to years). The patient must also be told that they are not causing any damage by using the limb, but rather that the affected part must be used as much as possible (which means that pain must sometimes be tolerated).

DOs and DON'Ts of Reflex Sympathetic Dystrophy

DO prescribe a daily set of exercises to stretch and strengthen the affected muscles and consult a rheumatologist if other therapies are being considered.

DO emphasize to the patient that in the late stage of the disease, only continued use of the affected region will help, and continuing work is beneficial.

DON'T use corticosteroids when swelling is no longer present, and do not use them for more than a few weeks at most. They are useful for the swelling and pain early on, but not afterward.

DON'T immobilize a patient with reflex sympathetic dystrophy.

DON'T prescribe narcotics or benzodiazepines.

DON'T confuse this with one of the chronic pain syndromes (note objective swelling and objective radiographic findings).

Section 5 – Outside the algorithm

Osteoporosis

Osteoporosis is a common disease, particularly in post-menopausal women. It is true that the vast majority of women will never suffer from an osteoporotic fracture even while having lower bone density than normal subjects. Nevertheless, this is somewhat unpredictable, and there are enough individuals who do suffer fractures, that prevention is considered to be worthwhile as long as it is carried out in a logical, cost-effective fashion with awareness of all the factors that modify risk for osteoporotic fractures, and the risks of therapies used for osteoporosis.

The most common fractures are Colles' fractures of the forearm, which for the most part heal well and do not cause significant disability. Vertebral fractures can be very painful, and may result in kyphosis. If enough fractures occur, the kyphosis becomes significant to the point where the lower rib cage descends towards the pelvis, producing a restrictive lung defect. Hip fractures have the highest morbidity, with 20–30% mortality in the first year, and usually an incomplete return to the previous level of function. All of these fractures may occur with minor trauma, and quite unpredictably.

There are still a number of unanswered questions from studies of osteoporosis. The group most likely to experience hip fractures includes women over the age of 65 years. Yet, the studies done to demonstrate prospectively a reduction in hip fracture incidence with therapy have very few patients in this age group. So while they do show benefit in the population studied, this population does not entirely include the subgroup of women most likely to have hip fractures.

It is also clear that the vast majority of studies use bone density measurements as the marker for whether or not a therapy is effective. It is assumed that an increase in bone density or prevention of its decrease is equivalent to a reduction in actual fractures. One must recall that we cannot supplant a reduction in a risk factor for a reduction in the incidence of fractures themselves. While a low bone density does translate into an increased incidence of fractures, the vast majority of patients with lower than normal bone density will never have a fracture. Thus, there are factors other than bone density which determine fracture incidence. These include falls, and changes in the 'architecture' of bone which may affect how well bone responds to stress. We do not have a good measure of these two factors.

We also do not have much information as to how patients with either multiple fractures, over the age of 65 years, or co-morbidity from other chronic diseases might respond to some of the therapies usually studied in healthier and younger patients.

Finally, there is an argument that estrogens are the treatment of choice for osteoporosis because they have a beneficial effect in reducing the incidence of cardiovascular disease. The data arguing for the cardiovascular benefits is not complete yet, as there are no prospective, randomized, double-blind, placebo-controlled studies to date.

Studies with calcitonin are not long enough, are too small, have methodologic faults, or lack appropriate clinical end points of fracture rather than just bone density. There is increasing good data about biphosphonates, although there are still methodologic faults in those studies. Biphosphonates are being used more often, however, because of this recent data.

As for when to order bone density measurements, there is a reasonable argument that in the light of health care cost restrictions, a bone density measurement is not likely to alter management and may not be cost-effective if ordered routinely. Whether the patient's bone density is normal or below normal will not, for example, alter the decision to offer a post-menopausal woman estrogen therapy. Some recommend routine serum calcium, phosphate, alkaline phosphatase, and 25–hydroxy-vitamin D levels in all patients. In older patients with a fracture, serum electropheresis is sometimes ordered to rule out multiple myeloma. One must weigh the costs of routine studies against the likelihood of detecting diseases such as osteomalacia (vitamin D deficiency), Paget's disease, etc. *Table 5.7* shows the results of these studies in each disease.

Table 5.7 Laboratory findings in metabolic bone disease

Disease	Serum calcium	Serum phosphate	Alkaline phosphatase	Vitamin D	Parathyroid hormone
Osteoporosis	N	N	N	N	N
Osteomalacia[a]	Low	Low	High	Low	High
Renal disease	Low	High	High	N	High
Primary hyper-parathyroidism	High	Low	N	N	Very high
Paget's disease	N	N	Very high	N	N

[a] This refers to osteomalacia due to nutritional vitamin D deficiency in the form of decreased sunlight exposure, malnourishment, or malabsorption.

Despite the limitations in our knowledge, it is important to use what information we do have in managing the patient with osteoporosis. The initial management of osteoporosis must address all reversible risk factors. One should specifically enquire about falls, provide a safer home environment, canes, walkers, education about avoiding icy surfaces, and look for other medical causes of falls. The patient should stop smoking and stop drinking alcohol. Although studies showing that exercise prevents osteoporosis and fractures are often flawed, exercise has beneficial effects on heart and lung disease, obesity, maintenance of muscle strength, agility (which might prevent falls), and quality of life. Patients should be advised to engage in an exercise program that is as active as they are capable (from simply daily walks to aerobics, etc.).

Risk factors for osteoporosis

The diagnosis of an acute osteoporotic fracture as a cause for back pain is important since calcitonin (see below) may be effective in relieving the pain of an acute fracture within days. It may be difficult to make this diagnosis, however. If a patient presents with back pain and an X-ray shows a fracture, one does not know for certain if that fracture is new or old. One way to address this is to order a bone scan. If the bone scan is negative, then this fracture is old. If it is positive, it is not entirely helpful because a bone scan may remain positive for several months after a fracture has occurred.

Table 5.8   Risk factors for osteoporosis

Smoking
Immobilization
Alcohol use
Endocrine
      Hyperthyroidism
      Cushing's syndrome
      Androgen loss
      Menopause (natural or surgical)

Falls
      Visual diseases (glaucoma, cataracts, refractive errors)
      Postural hypotension
      Muscle weakness (disuses, myopathy)
      Environmental (bathtubs, stairs)
      Cardiac (syncope, bradycardia, aortic stenosis)
      Arthritis
      Neurologic (Parkinson's, multiple sclerosis, previous strokes)

Calcium deficiency
      Dietary
      Malabsorption
      Losses in renal disease

Vitamin D deficiency
      Decreased exposure to sunlight
      Renal disease
      Anticonvulsants

Drugs
      Corticosteroids
      Cyclosporine
      Chronic heparin

If one suspects an acute fracture has occurred, because of acute, localized verte-bral pain and clear risk factors for a fracture (like a patient on corticosteroids), but the X-ray is normal, a bone scan should be performed. This will be posi-tive before the X-ray will (it may take 2 weeks for a fracture to be evident on X-ray). If the bone scan is negative, a fracture is ruled out.

Remember that osteoporosis is not painful unless a fracture has occurred. Patients are sometimes told that their back pain is due to osteoporosis, when this is often not the case.

Drug therapy

Calcium
There is still considerable debate about the role of dietary calcium in preventing bone loss or treating osteoporosis. There is no reason to expect very high calcium intake will increase already decreased bone mass. Nevertheless, most current recommendations advise that adult women have 800 mg qd of elemental calcium in their diet. This can be obtained by foods in most cases (e.g. 750 ml milk, three cups of dark green vegetables, 100 g of cheese). In cases where the patient does not want or cannot tolerate these calcium sources, supplements may be used. It is often difficult to expect higher nutritional intake, since women often have concerns about excess calories and fat intake that accompanies some foods with high calcium content.

In general, there is no good evidence that one form of supplement is better than another, although calcium carbonate may be less well absorbed in elderly women. The amount of the supplement prescribed depends on an assessment of dietary intake, so that the total intake is 800 mg qd in pre-menopausal women, and 1500 mg qd in post-menopausal women (the need for higher intake in this latter group is not proven, but commonly recommended). The physician should be aware that high calcium intake can sometimes be associated with constipa-tion, or renal stones (in patients with pre-existing hypercalciuria).

Vitamin D
Adequate vitamin D levels can be tested for by measuring the level of 25–hydroxy-vitamin D. If this is abnormal, vitamin D supplements are neces-sary. There is an increasing tendency to use vitamin D routinely in osteoporosis, although there is limited data on its ability to independently alter fracture incidence. About 400–1000 units per day is usually prescribed. Patients on anti-convulsants may benefit from vitamin D supplements because these drugs interfere with production of vitamin D in the skin.

Some patients with osteoporosis have hypercalciuria (> 240 mg in 24 h), and some recommend that if this is present, the patient be given hydrochloroth-iazide 25 mg bid to reduce calcium loss in the urine, which may worsen with vitamin D therapy. The benefit of doing this has not been proven, and one must be aware of the adverse effects due to hydrochlorothiazide therapy (hypercalcemia and hypokalemia).

Also, if a patient is on vitamin D therapy and becomes immobilized, it is wise to hold the vitamin D therapy until they are mobilized, as hypercalcemia may otherwise occur.

Hormones
Estrogen is the most common therapy. The advantages of hormonal therapy are prevention of Colles' and vertebral fractures (possibly hip fractures), possible decrease in cardiovascular disease, and relief of post-menopausal symptoms such as irritability, hot flushes, headaches, and dyspareunia. The disadvantages include the slightly higher risk of breast and endometrial carcinoma. It is likely that deep venous thrombosis is not a risk, since the doses of estrogen in oral contraceptives (which are associated with deep venous thrombosis) are much higher. The risk of endometrial carcinoma can be minimized by appropriate use of progesterone in combination with estrogen therapy, although it is not clear whether cardiac benefits occur in the face of progesterone. The risk of breast cancer is small, but patients who have had breast cancer in the past should never be on estrogens, and those with a positive family history should probably not as well.

The use of estrogens with progesterone (10 mg a day for last 10 days each month, withdrawing the estrogen) is associated with a return of menstrual periods, which many woman would prefer not to have. The options are to do one of the following:

1. Accept that menstrual periods will return;

2. Estrogen and progesterone (medroxyprogesterone 2.5–5.0 mg qd) continuously, which avoids menstrual periods;

3. Estrogen continuously and progesterone (10 mg for the last 10 days of each month) which leads to minor spotting for the first 4 months, and not after that; or

4. Estrogen continuously, then withdraw it every three months, using progesterone (10 mg qd for 10 days) to lead to menses every 3 months.

The optimal number of years of therapy is not known (but it is generally given for more than 5 years). It may not be cost effective to give 20 years of therapy and the long-term effects of this duration are not well studied.

Estrogen can be prescribed as conjugated estrogen 0.625 mg po qd, as a patch 50 μg twice weekly, or as estradiol 1–2 mg qd.

Hypertension, and hypertriglyceridemia may occur, both of which resolve within a few weeks if the drug is discontinued. Unexplained vaginal bleeding and hepatitis are contra-indications to starting therapy. Patients should have annual mammograms.

Calcitonin

Calcitonin is prescribed as 50–100 units sc qd, or intranasal. The best dose is unknown. The adverse effects include nausea or flushing, and the drug is costly. A particularly unique quality of calcitonin is that it can often be remarkably effective in relieving the pain of an acute osteoporotic vertebral fracture with just a few days of therapy. (Usually most vertebral fractures are symptomatic for six weeks otherwise.) Calcitonin is also sometimes used if a patient has failed therapy with etidronate (ongoing fractures or worsening bone density).

Biphosphonates

Biphosphonates are less expensive than calcitonin. One may use etidronate (5 mg/kg qd) either 2 h before or after a meal (otherwise it is bound by gastric contents) taken for 2 week cycles every 3 months. Calcium intake of 1500 mg qd must be prescribed, but the calcium intake must be at least 2 h since the last dose of etidronate, otherwise it will bind the etidronate which will then not be absorbed. Some recommend not prescribing the calcium at all during the two-week period of etidronate use, although some patients may find this difficult to remember. Alternative biphosphonates include pamidronate and alendronate.

Despite insufficient data, biphosphonates are currently the recommended therapy or prevention for corticosteroid-induced osteoporosis. If a patient is going to be on corticosteroids for more than 1 year, this should be considered, using doses as outlined above, as should calcium and vitamin D therapy.

Fluoride

The studies done to date do not support the use of fluoride in the treatment of osteoporosis, but there is currently a study in progress that suggests that sodium fluoride 25 mg po bid taken with calcium may be effective and safe. Higher doses than this are associated with adverse effects and an actual increase in the rate of fractures. Most recommend that any patient currently on fluoride should have it discontinued until further data are available.

Case scenarios of osteoporosis

1. *A 25–year-old woman would like to know what she can do to prevent osteoporosis because her mother has osteoporosis* Complete a history looking for the risk factors listed above. Recommend moderate exercise (like regular walking, or any exercise which requires weight-bearing, done for 30–60 minutes three times per week), smoking cessation, avoidance of alcohol, and calcium intake of a least 800 mg qd. Check for drug-associated osteoporosis, due to chronic heparin use, oral corticosteroids, or anticonvulsants.

2. *A woman has entered menopause (natural, early, or surgical) and would like to prevent osteoporosis* Do a complete history and physical examination (including Pap smear and mammogram), focusing on the risk factors above. If no systemic diseases are discovered, no routine blood work is required. Some would choose to do a lumbar spine X-ray and bone density measurement, but these may not alter management.

   Educate about modifying risk factors, and recommend calcium intake 1500 mg qd. Supplement with calcium if needed, and consider vitamin D 400–1000 units qd.

   If the patient is willing to consider hormone therapy, determine if the uterus is present and whether or not patient has significant risk factors for breast carcinoma (personal or family history of breast carcinoma). If no uterus is present, and there is no concern about breast carcinoma, then prescribe estrogens alone. If the uterus is present, and there is no concern about breast carcinoma, then prescribe estrogen and progesterone together. If contraindications to estrogen use or the patient is concerned about breast carcinoma, then consider etidronate or calcitonin therapy.

3. *A woman with menopause and current evidence of fractures* Do a complete history and physical examination (including Pap smear and mammogram), focusing on the risk factors described above. Ask about weight loss, fever, night sweats, bone pain elsewhere, and known malignancy. Do a baseline lumbar spine X-ray (some osteoporotic fractures are entirely asymptomatic and may already be present). Consider investigation of fracture cause by ordering CBC, calcium, phosphate, parathyroid hormone, and 25–hydroxy-vitamin D tests, and serum electropheresis. Consider risk factors and investigation for breast or lung carcinoma with metastases.

   Educate the patient about modifying risk factors and exercise. Recommend calcium intake of 1500 mg qd, and consider vitamin D treatment. If fracture is acutely painful, consider calcitonin treatment for a few days to relieve pain. Consider hormone therapy, etidronate, or calcitonin as in Case 2 above.

4. *A 36-year-old asthmatic with chronic need for oral corticosteroids* Corticosteroid-induced osteoporosis is a difficult problem. Corticosteroids can produce fractures in young patients, and even at bone densities higher than what is normally considered at risk. (This supports the idea that bone density alone is not the only predictor of fracture.) The best intervention is prevention, or using the lowest doses possible for the shortest time. There are no studies which have reported the incidence of fractures to ascertain whether there are therapies that can prevent or treat corticosteroid-induced osteoporosis. (A study with alendronate is underway.) Alternate day dosing of the corticosteroid does not alter risk for osteoporosis. Inhaled cortico-

steroids are not generally of concern, although topical ones may be in those using large amounts for skin diseases.

Educate the patient about modifying risk factors as in Case 1, above. Assess their daily intake of calcium, and supplement this if needed to give 1500 mg qd total intake, and give vitamin D.

Do a lumbar spine X-ray. Use the lowest possible dose of prednisone, (prednisolone) or consider giving a steroid-sparing drug, if available, for the patient's disease. Consider etidronate therapy. If etidronate is used, the patient should probably remain on it for a few months after stopping corticosteroids, although there is no good data to support this.

DOs and DON'Ts of Osteoporosis

DO start therapy with education about modifying the risk factors for osteoporosis.

DO consider osteomalacia, Paget's disease, malignancy, and multiple myeloma in the patient with fractures.

DO avoid using corticosteroids in any patient unless their disease mandates it, and all other options have been tried.

DON'T ascribe a patient's back pain to osteoporosis unless you have evidence of a fracture. Even then, remember that mechanical back pain is a more common cause of back pain.

DON'T tell patients with chronic pain syndromes that the cause of their pain is osteoporosis.

Outside the algorithm

Section 5 – Outside the algorithm

Pediatric rheumatology

Rheumatic diseases in children are far less common than in adults. This, coupled with the fewer number of pathognomonic symptoms or signs in childhood rheumatic diseases makes early referral to a rheumatologist worthwhile. The task, then, is to decide when a rheumatic disease may be present, and therefore whether referral is warranted. To simplify this task, begin by considering whether or not the child with complaints in the limbs or spine has any of the following:

1. appears unwell;

2. fever (it follows that the assessment of a child with fever includes joint examination);

3. erythema over joints; or

4. joint swelling (in some cases, the swelling may be painless, but warrants investigation just the same).

If any of these exist, referral to a rheumatologist is reasonable. In all cases, careful ophthalmologic examination for scarring of the iris or cornea must be carried out, as anterior uveitis in juvenile arthritis may be asymptomatic initially. If abnormalities are found on ocular examination, refer to an ophthalmologist immediately, otherwise referral is recommended within a few weeks. The minimum investigations include a CBC with peripheral smear, ESR, renal function, tests for liver enzymes, blood cultures (if febrile), ANA test, RF test, and X-rays of the affected area.

In addition, there are some important differences between the etiology of childhood rheumatic complaints and those seen in adults, and some conditions specific to childhood that one should be aware of.

Sprains

Sprain due to trauma in children seldom causes symptoms that will last for more than 5 days. If it does, then either fracture, significant ligament or cartilage tear, or a nontraumatic etiology should be considered.

Back pain

Back pain lasting more than a few weeks in children should be thoroughly investigated (X-ray, bone scan, and possibly CT scan or MRI), with referral. Causes of back pain in children and some methods for diagnosis are shown in *Table 5.9*.

Table 5.9 The etiology of back pain in children

Trauma
    Fracture (X-ray)
    Spondylosis/spondylolisthesis (X-ray)
    Hematoma (bone scan, CT or MRI)

Infection
    Vertebral or sacroiliac osteomyelitis (bone scan, CT or MRI, CT-guided aspiration)
    Discitis (X-ray finding of blurred vertebral end-plate margin, bone scan, CT-guided aspiration)

Inflammatory
    Seronegative spondyloarthropathy (X-ray, bone scan)
    Scheuermann's disease (painful kyphosis in adolescence and X-ray)

Tumor (bone scan, CT or MRI)

Nonrheumatic
    Pyelonephritis
    Renal tumor
    Renal stone

Limp

Limp must always be investigated and/or generate referral. Causes of limp in children and some methods for diagnosis are shown in *Table 5.10*. Joint examination in children should include checking for limb length discrepancy.

Growing pains

Growing pains can only be diagnosed if the child has nocturnal-only symptoms of lower limb pain (behind the knee or shins). Any other pattern warrants a search for another diagnosis.

Muscle weakness

Muscle weakness is more difficult to detect and grade in young children. Suspicious signs of myopathy include:

1. Child who was walking is refusing to do so

2. Child must roll on to side first to sit up

3. Child cannot stand on tip toes or stand from squatting

Table 5.10 The etiology of limp in children

Trauma
     Fracture of limb, back, or pelvis (X-ray)
     Meniscal injury (arthrogram, MRI)
     Loose body in knee (X-ray, arthrogram, or MRI)
     Avulsion fractures at tibial tuberosity, or Achilles insertion (X-ray, bone scan)

Infection
     Septic arthritis (aspiration)
     Vertebral or sacroiliac osteomyelitis (bone scan, CT or MRI, CT-guided aspiration)
     Discitis (X-ray finding of blurred vertebral end-plate margin, bone scan, CT-guided
        aspiration)

Inflammatory
     Spondyloarthropathy (X-ray, bone scan)
     Juvenile arthritis (diagnosis of exclusion)
     Polymyositis/dermatomyositis (CK, muscle biopsy)

Tumor (bone scan, CT or MRI)

Miscellaneous
     Legg-Perthes disease (X-ray, CT or MRI)
     Hypermobility syndrome (see below)
     Arch collapse

4. Gower's sign – child uses hands along thighs to get to a standing position

5. Wide-base gait (where previously normal)

6. Significant head lag when lifting child from supine to sitting position (after 4 months of age)

(See polymyositis in previous sections)

Hypermobility syndrome

Hypermobility may produce symptoms of pain referable to the low back, hip, knee, wrist and hand, and ankle and foot. The diagnostic criteria for hypermobility are:

1. thumb abducts passively to touch forearm;

2. fingers extend passively beyond 90°;

3. elbows extend passively beyond 10°;

4. knees extend passively beyond 10°;

5. with knees straight, child can bend and place palms on floor.

This syndrome places individuals at risk for overuse injuries including tendinitis, muscle tears, ligament tears, back pain, arch collapse, and recurrent joint dislocation.

Table 5.11 Differential diagnosis of spine or limb pain in children

Diagnostic clue	Possible diagnosis	Investigation
Any of fever, very painful joint, erythema	Septic arthritis Osteomyelitis	Aspiration for Gram stain and culture, bone scan
Any of sore throat, known *Strep.* throat, pericardial rub, nodules, rash, movement disorder	Rheumatic fever	ESR, throat swab, anti-streptolysin-O titre, echocardiogram
Recent immunization	Post-immunization arthralgias	
Preceding viral illness	Post-viral arthritis Consider Lyme disease	
Chronic cough, known TB risk factor	Tuberculous septic arthritis	Mantoux, aspiration for TB staining Synovial biopsy for TB if above negative
Preceding trauma	Fracture Intra-articular bleeding Septic arthritis from penetrating injury Avulsion fractures	X-ray Aspiration, X-ray, bone scan Aspiration X-ray, bone scan
Any of iritis, psoriasis, nail pitting, low back pain, limited back range of motion, heel pain	Spondyloarthropathy	X-ray, bone scan
Preceding upper respiratory or diarrheal illness, conjunctivitis, or dysuria	Reactive arthritis	Exclude other causes of arthritis
Chronic bloody diarrhea	Inflammatory bowel disease	Endoscopy X-ray, bone scan
Pain over bones	Malignancy Fracture Osteoid osteoma Osteomyelitis	X-ray, bone scan
Point-specific tenderness over tarsal navicular bone, carpal lunate, 2nd or 3rd metatarsal head	Osteonecrosis	X-ray, bone scan
Erythema migrans[a], meningitis, polyneuropathy, cranial neuropathy, or cardiac dysrhythmias	Lyme disease[b]	Lyme serology
Elbow pain, without swelling	Nursemaid's elbow[c] (elbow joint dislocation)	Reduce dislocation
Multiple fractures (skull, ribs, femur) Skin bruising, abrasions, burns	Child abuse	Police

[a] Present in 60% of cases, this rash has a central clearing area with rapidly expanding lesions, appearing in varied sites, and disappearing in weeks to months.
[b] Endemic areas are Lake Erie in Canada, the Northeast and west coast, and the upper Midwest of the United States, and Central Europe.
[c] Occurs when a small child is pulled forcefully by the hand or wrist with the elbow extended. This may dislocate the joint and the child may complain of pain near the elbow, or simply stop using the arm. The arm will be pronated and the elbow held in flexion. Correct it by placing the thumb of one hand on the radial head, fully flex the elbow, and then supinate it.

Management

Arthralgias may be difficult to manage (even with analgesics), and most recommend muscle strengthening exercises involving the back extensors, forearm flexors, and hamstrings. Arch supports may be helpful. Otherwise, ligament tears, muscle tears, and tendinitis are given standard therapy.

Thus, through consideration of the five key signs that referral is needed, and by recognizing the specific issues regarding trauma, back pain, limp, growing pains, muscle weakness, and hypermobility, a diagnosis or need for referral will become apparent.

Beyond this, clues to some specific causes of arthritis or arthralgias are shown in *Table 5.11*. It is important to consider this list before ever concluding that the diagnosis is juvenile arthritis (and indeed, such a diagnosis should be confirmed by a rheumatologist). The child with juvenile chronic arthritis, spondyloarthropathy, myopathy, SLE, and vasculitis should be co-managed with a rheumatologist. The specifics of such management in children is beyond the intended purpose of this book.

Case scenarios of juvenile arthritis

The important considerations in the diagnosis and management of juvenile arthritis are that one must consider the many other diagnostic possibilities as described above, wait at least 8 weeks before making a diagnosis of juvenile chronic arthritis (since there are short-lived, unexplained inflammatory episodes, such as reactive arthritis, which may persist for up to this time), and should consider obtaining assistance from a rheumatologist. If a diagnosis of juvenile arthritis is considered, careful examination of the cornea and iris for scarring from chronic uveitis is necessary. In addition, in patients with a diagnosis of juvenile arthritis, regular assessment by an opthalmologist and rheumatologist is generally recommended. The typical patterns of juvenile arthritis one should be aware of are pauciarticular onset (most common pattern), systemic-onset, and juvenile rheumatoid arthritis (rheumatoid factor positive polyarthritis).

Pauciarticular-onset juvenile chronic arthritis is characterized by involvement of four joints, or fewer, in the first 6 months, with girls less than 6 years old being most often affected, a predilection for the knees, ankles, and wrists, presence of chronic anterior uveitis, and typically negative rheumatoid factor, normal or slightly elevated ESR, and positive ANA.

Systemic-onset juvenile chronic arthritis (Still's disease) is characterized by prominent extra-articular features including daily fever, an evanescent, pink, diffuse, myalgias, adenopathy, and sometimes hepatosplenomegaly, pleuritis, or pericarditis. There may be little or no arthritis at the onset, although arthralgias are often present. Anemia, leukocytosis, thrombocytosis, high ESR, negative rheumatoid factor, and negative ANA are typical. There is, of course, a wide differential diagnosis, especially in those patients without arthrotis initially.

Finally, polyarticular, and rheumatoid factor-positive juvenile arthritis is characterized by features typical of adult rheumatoid arthritis, with erosive disease in many cases, requiring similar therapy as in adults.

Case 1. A 4-year-old boy has a 2 week history of a swollen, mildly painful right ankle. There is no morning stiffness, fever, prior trauma, tavel to endemic areas, or family history positive for arthritis, iritis, psoriasis, or inflammatory bowel disease. There was no antecedent evidence of pharyngitis or other infections. Physical examination reveals a well-looking child with effusion of the ankle, normal joint range of motion, normal spine examination, and no other abnormal joints. The pupils and cornea reveal no evidence of scarring. Cardiovascular examination is normal, and there is no rash or subcutaneous nodules.

The most likely diagnoses are either reactive arthritis (sometimes a clear antecedent infection is not identified) or pauciarticular juvenile chronic arthritis. The patient is started in an NSAID. The patient is referred to an ophthalmologist for further examination, and to a rheumatologist. CBC, ESR, urinalysis, and rheumatoid factor are negative, while ANA titer is 1:160.

The normal ESR makes reactive arthritis unlikely, and so the diagnosis of chronic pauciarticular onset juvenile arthritis is made, presuming that the duration of symptoms will be at least 6–8 weeks. The ophthalmologist makes recommendations for further ocular examinations and treatment if needed, and a rheumatologist will advise on treatment if NSAIDs are ineffective.

Case 2. A 5-year-old boy develops the acute onset of high fever, rash, anorexia, malaise, and diffuse arthralgias and myalgias, with no other symptoms to suggest a specific focus of infection. He has no significant travel history, drug use, known illness contacts or weight loss.

Examination reveals an ill-looking boy, in mild discomfort, febrile, with pink, macular rash on his trunk only. There is no synovitis, nodules, adenopathy, abdominal organomegaly, pharyngitis, and abnormalities on the cardiovascular examination (except tachycardia in keeping with the fever) or chest examination. There is no neck stiffness or neurologic abnormalities.

The differential is wide, and investigations include CBC, ESR, ANA, rheumatoid factor, renal function, liver enzymes, hepatic function, chest X-ray, ECG, blood cultures, throat swab, urinalysis and culture, abdominal and pelvic ultrasound, and ocular examination. Broad spectrum antibiotics are started, pending culture results.

The only positive investigations are leucocytosis, thrombocytosis, and high ESR. A lumbar puncture is performed, and after 48 hours with cerebrospinal and other cultures negative, antibiotics are stopped. Systemic-onset juvenile arthritis is considered in light of other negative findings, and the patient responds to an NSAID.

Case 3. A 10-year-old girl develops the gradual onset of pain and swelling in multiple joints of the hands, and in the feet and both knees over a 6 week period. There is marked morning stiffness, no fever, no pack pain, no rash, no travel to endemic areas for Lyme disease, or family history positive for arthritis, iritis, psoriasis, or inflammatory bowel disease. There was no antecedent evidence of pharyngitis or other infections. Physical examination reveals synovitis of a number of MCP and PIP joints of the hands, as well as both knees and the MTP joints of the feet. There is normal spine examination, no other abnormal joints, no rash, no adenopathy, no pharyngitis or oral lesions, no abdominal organomegaly, and no nodules. The pupils and cornea reveal no evidence of scarring. Cardiovascular examination is normal.

The most likely diagnosis is juvenile rheumatoid arthritis. The patient is started on an NSAID, and referred to a rheumatologist. Laboratory findings include mild normocytic anemia, normal white cell count, thrombocytosis, elevated ESR, negative ANA, positive rheumatoid factor, normal urinalysis, and normal X-rays (other than soft-tissue swelling). The rheumatologist recommends starting gold therapy.

DOs and DON'Ts of Pediatric Rheumatology

DO have a rheumatologist involved early in the child with a rheumatic complaint.

DO complete a joint and spine examination in the child with fever.

DO consider child abuse if there are multiple fractures involving ribs, skull, or femur, and skin abrasions, bruises, or burns.

DO refer and/or thoroughly investigate back pain and limp.

DO have X-rays taken and reviewed in a center with experience in pediatric radiology.

DO suspect septic arthritis if fever, inability to move joint, erythema, or high ESR are present.

DO ask about travel history and TB risk factors.

DO remember that patellofemoral syndrome is a common cause of knee pain in teenagers.

DO remember to prescribe drug dosages for children according to recommendations (usually by the child's weight).

DON'T accept sprain as the cause of symptoms lasting more than 5 days. Investigate further.

DON'T diagnose chronic pain syndrome in a child unless confirmed by a rheumatologist.

DON'T diagnose juvenile arthritis unless confirmed by a rheumatologist.

DON'T treat septic arthritis with antibiotics alone. Drainage is necessary.

Section 6 – Treatment

Drug therapy

It is generally recommended that patients with chronic rheumatic diseases receive pneumovaccine and yearly influenza vaccine.

Nonsteroidal anti-inflammatory drugs (NSAIDs)

The term NSAID conventionally refers to those drugs whose mechanism is interference with arachidonic acid metabolism. There are numerous classes of NSAIDs (*Table 6.1*), and some believe that each class may demonstrate effectiveness where others have failed. Knowledge of the different classes is used in some patients to plan a series of NSAID choices to be tried next, before abandoning this group of drugs as primary therapy. Still others believe patients who fail to respond to one NSAID class will not have significant benefit from others.

NSAIDs are used for both their anti-inflammatory and analgesic properties, the latter tending to require lower doses. About 650 mg of ASA, 50 mg of indomethacin, 650 mg of acetaminophen (paracetamol), and 30 mg of codeine are relatively equal in analgesic efficacy. For their anti-inflammatory benefit, it is recommended that NSAIDs be used regularly until a stable clinical state is reached, or the need for additional therapy is evident.

Indomethacin seems to be among the most potent, but is also associated with a higher incidence of adverse effects. Although some conditions seem to respond to certain NSAID classes, there are few well performed, appropriate studies to verify this and it is not easy to predict which class will be the best for the individual patient. Although NSAIDs often give relief of symptoms in a few days, it may take 2 to 4 weeks before a complete, stable response occurs. Most appropriate trials of NSAIDs should be of this duration before changing classes or introducing new therapy. There is no evidence that combinations of NSAIDs are better than monotherapy, and adverse effects may be increased with combinations.

There are numerous adverse effects to NSAIDs, but the most important are renal and gastrointestinal toxicity. Renal insufficiency usually occurs within 3 to 7 days of initiating therapy, and risk factors for this complication include increased age,

Table 6.1 NSAID classes and dosages in rheumatoid arthritis[a]

NSAID	Dose
Salsalate (Disalcid®)	1500 mg bid
Trisalicylate (Trilisate®)	1000 mg bid–tid
Acetylsalicylic acid (Aspirin®)	650–975 mg qid
Diflunisal (Dolobid®)	250–500 mg bid
Sulfinpyrazone (Salazopyrin®)	500 mg qid
Indomethacin (Indocid®)	50 mg tid
Sulindac (Clinoril®)	150–200 mg bid
Tolmetin (Tolectin®)	400–600 mg tid
Naproxen (Naprosyn®)	250–500 mg bid
Ibuprofen (Motrin®)	800 mg tid–qid
Ketoprofen (Orudis®)	50 mg tid–qid
Flurbiprofen (Ansaid®)	50 mg tid–qid
Fenoprofen (Nalfon®)	600 mg tid–qid
Tiaprofenic acid (Surgam®)	200–300 mg tid
Diclofenac (Voltaren®)	50 mg tid–qid
Mefenamic acid(Ponstan®)	250 mg qid
Floctafenine (Idarac®)	200–400 mg tid
Tenoxicam (Mobiflex®)	20 mg qd
Piroxicam (Feldene®)	20 mg qd
Nabumetone (Relafen®)	1–2 g qd

[a] Not all trade names are given, merely examples.

diabetes, hypertension, and co-incident use of drugs which alter renal blood flow (e.g. angiotensin converting enzyme inhibitors). NSAIDs are best avoided or used under close supervision in patients with renal insufficiency. The non-acetylated salicylates, salsalate and trisalicylate may be safe in renal disease.

Gastrointestinal side-effects are the most common. The majority of symptoms include abdominal pain, nausea, and dyspepsia. These do not, unfortunately, correlate well with the development of the more serious complications such as gastric or duodenal ulcers. In fact, some patients will have gastrointestinal bleeds without prior warning symptoms. Indomethacin and noncoated ASA may be the most frequent offenders, whereas enteric coded ASA may be the least, the other NSAID classes being intermediate. Patients over 65 years of age seem to be most at risk for bleeds. Although suppository forms are available for some NSAIDs, these do not confer protection from gastrointestinal complications, and are not necessarily better tolerated than oral forms.

Cytoprotection with misoprostol should be offered to any patient taking NSAIDs who is at higher risk for a complication (either over the age of 65 years, or who has had a previous bleed or perforation from NSAIDs). Until recently, there were no studies that assessed the efficacy of cytoprotective therapy in reducing the incidence of GI bleeds, perforation, or death (only incidence of endoscopic lesions were studied). There has now been, however, a large prospective study that shows misoprostol 200 μg bid with an NSAID reduces complications, and that it is cost-effective to routinely prescribe it to the two types of patients above. One cannot use symptoms to identify those who need cytoprotection, since the correlation with symptoms is poor, and therefore all patients in this higher risk group must be offered prophylaxis routinely. In order to lessen the symptoms of diarrhea from misoprostol, the drug should be taken with a meal. The patient should be aware that this side-effect usually resolves within 3 days, and one can use 100 μg bid for about one week to build tolerance if diarrhea occurs.

Hypersensitivity may occur with all NSAIDs, and in particular one should be cautious in those who have serious allergies to ASA, especially people with asthma who develop bronchospasm with ASA use.

The best way to avoid NSAID associated complications is to avoid NSAIDs.

DOs and DON'Ts of NSAIDs

DO consider renal dysfunction before placing an elderly patient on an NSAID, checking their renal function at some point, and know that NSAIDs can cause hyperkalemia and fluid overload.

DO remember that if one NSAID was ineffective, one from another class may work.

DO tell the patient that it may take 2–4 weeks for good NSAID effect.

DO start with lower doses in the elderly, and consider using once-a-day NSAIDs.

DON'T assume that because the patient has been given a 'cytoprotective' agent that they can never have a GI bleed.

Systemic corticosteroids

Since their introduction in the form of cortisone in the 1950s, corticosteroids have been used for the treatment of many rheumatic diseases (*Table 6.2*). They have also been associated with a great number of adverse effects and are best used judiciously in chronic diseases because of this.

Table 6.2 Systemic corticosteroids used in rheumatic diseases

Drug	Milligram equivalents
Dexamethasone	0.75
Triamcinolone	4
Methylprednisolone	4
Prednisone (prednisolone)	5
Hydrocortisone	20
Cortisone	25

Table 6.3 Adverse effects of corticosteroids

General
    Anxiety, tremor, palpitations
    Weight gain
    Impaired wound healing
    Susceptibility to infections
    Psychosis
    Insomnia
    (?)Increased risk for NSAID gastropathy

Musculoskeletal
    Osteoporosis
    Myopathy
    Avascular necrosis

Cardiovascular
    Salt retention
    Hypertension

Endocrine
    Hyperglycemia
    Hyperlipidemia
    Pituitary suppression

Skin
    Atrophy
    Bruising
    Acne

Ophthalmic
    Glaucoma
    Cataracts

Acutely, these drugs may cause euphoria, tremulousness, confusion, psychosis, hypertension, and salt retention. In the long term, they may cause osteoporosis, avascular necrosis, skin atrophy, cataracts, poor wound healing, and predisposition to infections, to name a few (see *Table 6.3*). Local injections of corticosteroid have adverse effects such as an initial aggravation of inflammation for 24–48 h post-injection, and, uncommonly, skin depigmentation at the site of injection if it was delivered too superficially.

There are, of course, specific diseases for which systemic corticosteroids are definitely indicated. Here, the aim is to control the disease and slowly taper the corticosteroid according to clinical and laboratory measures, until the smallest effective dose is reached or the drug is discontinued altogether.

There is no standard way of tapering corticosteroids, since some conditions allow for a relatively rapid taper (weeks), while others are tapered over several months. Clinical experience with the diseases is often the most useful guide, as is simply trial and error.

DOs and DON'Ts of Corticosteroids

DON'T prescribe oral corticosteroids for osteoarthritis, chronic pain syndromes, or vague aches and pains.

DON'T prescribe corticosteroids because 'all else has failed'. Consult a rheumatologist for their opinion.

Local corticosteroids

The use of corticosteroid injections for the treatment of soft-tissue rheumatism is advocated by some, and opposed by others. At one extreme, it is probably incorrect simply to inject tender sites and send the patient away with no recommendations for preventing further injury, or for using physiotherapy to deal with the complications of such inflammatory conditions (like disuse muscle atrophy and immobility) and prevent future episodes. At the other extreme, some conditions remove the patient from their work environment and an attempt to treat the patient with physiotherapy alone may be successful, but take weeks. A balanced approach must be taken.

Most would agree that when an individual has been carrying out a repetitive activity (like painting a house for 3 days) and develops tendinitis, simply the fact that they have stopped the activity, and the use of physiotherapy is likely to lead to fairly prompt resolution. Most also agree that there is less tendency for athletes to be given injections, since the athlete may return to activity with physiotherapy exercises which lead to a better state of conditioning for the involved part. On the other hand, patients with rheumatoid arthritis often develop tendinitis even though they are on a regular exercise program, and despite physiotherapy. These patients do well with corticosteroid injections in combination with ongoing physiotherapy.

The physician must consider the type of patient he or she encounters, and develop an approach on this basis. Further comments regarding corticosteroid injections are to be found in Appendix 3.

Slow-acting drugs for rheumatoid arthritis

This group of drugs are referred to by many terms, including disease-modifying, or second-line. Slow-acting is used here because their slow onset of clinical benefit is well known, whereas the capacity to modify rheumatoid arthritis (in terms of joint damage) remains unproven, and second-line suggests something else should be prescribed first. There is a greater tendency to introduce these drugs earlier in the disease course in the hopes of limiting joint destruction. Thus, when one is confident that the diagnosis is rheumatoid arthritis (i.e. meets diagnostic criteria), a slow-acting anti-rheumatic drug should be started.

The exact mechanism of these drugs is not fully understood, although many effects on the immune system have been demonstrated. Because of the slow action of these drugs, temporizing measures such as NSAIDs, physiotherapy, and intra-articular corticosteroid injections are needed. The drugs, their important adverse effects, monitoring protocols, and costs are listed in *Table 6.4.* (Dosages provided are for adults.)

Rheumatologists often differ on which slow-acting anti-rheumatic drug they would choose first, how they might proceed to other choices, and how they might combine some of the drugs. It is very important to inform the patients of adverse effects, and the need for compliance with toxicity monitoring.

If there are adverse effects due to a slow-acting anti-rheumatic drug that cannot be corrected by temporarily changing the dose, holding a dose, or countermeasures, one should not simply stop the drug indefinitely and hope the patient will stay in remission indefinitely. They will not, and when their arthritis recurs, the whole process of patiently waiting for a new drug to work will have to be carried out. If one is in this situation of needing to stop therapy, contact a rheumatologist for advice, or introduce a new drug within a few weeks, while the patient is still well.

Once a patient has achieved a response with a given drug and is tolerating it, they should never stop the drug. Some patients do so well that they one day feel they no longer need their drug therapy. If they stop their therapy, the symptoms will flare, though it may take months, or a year. It will take as much time (often longer) to achieve remission again. **Unless a problem arises, never stop a slow-acting drug that is working.**

Gold compounds

Gold therapy may be oral or parenteral (IM). The two different forms may act by different mechanisms, so that failure of therapeutic effect with one form does not preclude successful therapy with the alternate form. Gold is successful in 50–70% of patients with rheumatoid arthritis.

The parenteral forms are sodium aurothiomalate (Myochrysine®) and aurothioglucose (Solganal®). The oral form is auranofin (Ridaura®).

Table 6.4 The slow-acting anti-rheumatic drugs in rheumatoid arthritis

Drug	Adverse effects	Monitoring	Cost in first 6 months ($)[a]	Annual ($)[a]
Gold (oral)	Diarrhea, abdominal pain, nausea Dermatitis, pruritus, stomatitis Proteinuria Leukopenia, thrombocytopenia	Monthly CBC, urinalysis	500	1000
Gold (IM)	Post-injection flushing Dermatitis, pruritus, stomatitis Proteinuria, nephrotic syndrome Leukopenia, thrombocytopenia Aplastic anemia (rare) Interstitial lung disease Bronchilitis obliterans (rare) Diarrhea, colitis	Weekly CBC, urinalysis for first 20 weeks, then every injection	900	700
Penicillamine	Anorexia, nausea Dermatitis, stomatitis Leukopenia, thrombocytopenia Aplatic anemia (rare) Proteinuria, nephrotic syndrome Bronchiolitis obliterans (rare)	Monthly CBC, urinalysis	600	1300
Methotrexate	Diarrhea, abdominal pain, nausea Dermatitis, pruritus, stomatitis Headache and memory impairment Cytopenias Elevated liver enzymes Interstitial lung disease Hepatic cirrhosis (rare)	Weekly CBC for 3 months then every 4 weeks Liver enzymes every 4–8 weeks	450	500
Anti-malarials	Diarrhea, abdominal pain, nausea Headache, irritability, insomnia Psychosis, nightmares Vestibular disturbances Dermatitis, psoriasis exacerbation Retinopathy, neuropathy Leukopenia	At least annual ophthalmology 150–300[b] exam		300–600
Sulfasalazine	Abdominal pain, nausea Dermatitis Leukopenia, thrombocytopenia Azoospermia	Monthly CBC to 3 months, then every few months	300	400

[a] Prices are based on average doses, costs to the patient from a dispensary, and include laboratory costs.
[b] The lower value is for chloroquine, the higher for hydroxychloroquine.

A trial of parenteral gold therapy entails administering a test dose of 25 mg to assess for post-injection reactions such as flushing, pruritus and hypotension. If the patient on parenteral gold develops post-injection flushing, pruritus, or arthralgias, one may try a repeat test dose in 1 week or try using the alternate parenteral preparation (i.e. change from Myochrysine® to Solganol® or vice versa). Since this reaction is uncommon, and may not be dose-related, some rheumatologists start patients at 50 mg routinely.

Then 50 mg IM weekly is given for 20 weeks (total dose equals 1000 mg). If the patient appears to have benefit after 20 weeks, with complete resolution of synovitis, and seems stable, one may try spacing injections to every 2 weeks. After another 3 months, if the disease remains controlled, injections may be spaced to every 3 weeks for another three months, then monthly. If a flare occurs during maintenance therapy, one may consider re-instituting weekly injections and then gradually returning to monthly maintenance. Alternatively, flares can be managed with NSAIDs and perhaps intra-articular corticosteroid injections. Sometimes both are necessary. If a patient does not respond after the first 20 weeks, a change in drug therapy is usually indicated.

Oral gold is little used in North America, but more so in Europe, though even there it is falling out of favour. It is given in doses of 6 mg qd (3 mg bid) for 6 months. If this is effective the patient will remain on this dose indefinitely. If not, or if a patient has a flare while on 6 mg qd, 9 mg qd may be tried for a few months. Oral gold has less toxicity than the parenteral form, but is probably less effective.

Prior to initiating gold therapy, one should obtain baseline urinalysis and CBC. This is checked 1–2 weeks initially to monitor for toxicity and then every 4–6 weeks.

Gold induced nephrotic syndrome is usually reversible, but might need corticosteroid therapy. The finding of greater than 1+ on a few consecutive occasions, is an indication for holding the patients next dose or doses, and if 24–h collection continues to show proteinuria of greater than 0.4 g qd, therapy should be stopped altogether.

It is also recommended that if the WBC count is less than $4.0 \times 10^9/l$ or platelet count less than $100 \times 10^9/l$, the next dose of gold be held, and the CBC repeated at that time instead. Persistent, borderline values are not usually worrisome to most rheumatologists, but it is worthwhile to ask their advice if this is occurring. Do not simply hold the gold injections indefinitely, because the patient will eventually flare. A plan of reinstituting therapy or changing drugs must be in place.

D-penicillamine

This drug may be as effective as gold, but also has a relatively high incidence of adverse effects and is slower acting than gold. The drug is started at 250 mg qd then increased in 4 weeks to 500 mg qd then after another 8 weeks 750 mg qd. Twelve weeks of 750 mg qd and no significant response is considered a failure of therapy. The drug does not necessarily have to be taken on an empty stomach without other drugs at the same time, although this is often stated. One should monitor CBC and urinalysis every 2–4 weeks, with the same recommendations as for gold. Allergy to penicillin is not a contra-indication to penicillamine.

Methotrexate

This drug has a more rapid onset than either gold or penicillamine therapy, and may have higher efficacy. It is usually started at 7.5–10 mg per week in either its oral or parenteral form. When given orally, the patient will take 7.5 mg on one day of the week (dose may be divided over a 24–h period), and not the other days. The patient must clearly understand that they cannot take it daily. Some prefer the IM or sc route because it documents compliance and avoids the inadvertent daily use of the oral form by the patient. The dose is increased by 2.5–5.0 mg in 4–8 weeks if no significant response. Further dosage increases can be made at 4–8 week intervals to a total dose of 25–35 mg per week. Above this dose, toxicity tends to limit its use, but some rheumatologists attempt these higher doses. If one is considering doses above 20 mg per week then it may be worthwhile to have a rheumatologist involved.

After 3 months one may try to reduce injections to every 2 weeks, but often this is unsuccessful, and weekly doses are needed. For the first 3 months one should have pre-injection CBC. If the total white count is less than 4.0, the subsequent dose should be held until a repeat CBC is done. Prior to starting therapy one should obtain baseline CBC, levels of blood urea nitrogen, creatinine, serum glutamic-oxaloacetic transaminase (SGOT), and albumin, and a chest X-ray. (Some include hepatitis serology as well.) For monitoring, in addition to weekly CBC, patients should have creatinine, SGOT, and albumin measured every 4–8 weeks.

Liver enzyme levels of tests are done every 4–8 weeks. Although elevated liver enzymes do not clearly predict liver cirrhosis (a rare event with less than a 6–8 g cumulative dose), it is generally recommended that the subsequent dosing be held or reduced until they normalize. Pre-therapy liver biopsy is not currently recommended by most rheumatologists in patients who do not have risk factors for chronic liver disease. Biopsy may be reasonable, however, in patients who have had abnormal liver enzymes in the past or who had a pretreatment history of significant alcohol intake. Patients should be warned not to drink alcohol while taking methotrexate. Remember that NSAIDs can cause elevated liver enzymes, and one should first consider discontinuing these before reducing the dose of methotrexate.

Pulmonary toxicity appears most often as hypersensitivity pneumonitis characterized by nonproductive cough, dyspnea, and fever. Bilateral pulmonary infiltrates develop, and fibrosis may eventually occur. Management includes stopping the methotrexate, confirming the diagnosis and looking for pulmonary infection (including opportunistic infections) by bronchoscopy, and beginning high-dose corticosteroids. Patients with significant pre-existing pulmonary disease are often not started on methotrexate because the occurrence of acute pneumonitis in such patients may be poorly tolerated.

Adverse effects of nausea and abdominal pain are often relieved by folic acid 1 mg or 5 mg qd. Leukopenia or thrombocytopenia often respond to holding one or two doses of methotrexate and/or by giving folic acid supplements for a few weeks. If patients continue to have nausea and abdominal pain despite folic acid, one may try folinic acid 2.5–5.0 mg, 24 h after the methotrexate dose. The response to CBC results should be the same as described above for gold.

Antimalarials

Hydroxychloroquine and chloroquine (the latter not available in the United States) have been used in a number of rheumatic diseases (particularly SLE). They are less effective in rheumatoid arthritis but are well tolerated and perhaps faster acting than gold. A trial of hydroxychloroquine is 400 mg qd for 6 months, after which the dose may be maintained there or reduced to 200 mg qd. Hydoxychloroquine is also used more frequently than chloroquine in the UK, although some rheumatologists in both Canada and the UK continue to use chloroquine, emphasizing that it is as effective, much less expensive, and that renal toxicity is minimized by careful monitoring. Chloroquine is generally prescribed as 250 mg qd for at least 6 months. Because of the rare adverse effect of retinopathy, an ophthalmological examination is obtained before initiating therapy and then every 6–12 months (typically 12 months is used). Chloroquine has been reported to produce retinopathy more often than hydroxychloroquine, and so strict monitoring is required, particularly at higher doses of chloroquine.

The safety of chloroquine in pregnancy is documented by the large number of cases of anti-malarial prophylaxis in pregnant women. The safety of hydroxy-chloroquine in pregnancy is supported to some extent by studies in pregnant systemic lupus erythematosus patients.

If early retinal toxicity is detected, the dosage could be reduced to half with repeat examination in 4–6 months. If the toxicity persists, or if more severe toxicity is detected (e.g. definite scotoma), antimalarial therapy should be discontinued.

Sulfasalazine

Sulfasalazine is 5–ASA covalently bound to sulfapyridine, the latter being the active moiety in rheumatoid arthritis. The benefits of sulfasalazine are that it generally acts faster than gold or penicillamine, with a better toxicity profile. There is a substantial emerging body of evidence that sulfasalazine is effective in psoriatic arthritis and ankylosing spondylitis. The most common adverse effects are nausea, abdominal pain, headache, and dizziness. These may be minimized by beginning at the dosage of 0.5 g bid, then increasing to 1.0 g bid 1–2 weeks later. The dose may be increased to 3.0 g qd if benefit is not significant after this time before concluding that there is a failure of therapy. The more serious adverse effects include cytopenias (up to 5%) which can occur at any time during therapy. Therefore, the CBC should be monitored every 4–6 weeks, with the guidelines as for penicillamine. Acute pneumonitis can occur (fever, cough, dyspnea) and requires drug cessation, and occasionally prednisone therapy after other causes have been ruled out. As well, liver enzymes may become elevated while on sulfasalazine, which may necessitate temporary withdrawal of the drug or dosage reduction.

Others

Combinations of the above drugs have been used by some rheumatologists quite successfully. There are few large studies on the use of other agents such as azathioprine, cyclophoshpamide, cyclosporin, or chlorambucil. These patients should be managed by a rheumatologist when introducing these drugs.

DOs and DON'Ts of Drug Therapy in Rheumatoid Arthritis

DO start a patient with rheumatoid arthritis on a slow-acting anti-rheumatic drug once the diagnosis is certain. Remember the symptoms and signs must be present for a minimum of 6 weeks.

DO educate the patient about the need for close monitoring of certain therapies with blood work and urinalysis, and check renal function, urinalysis, and CBC (and liver enzymes for methotrexate) before starting these drugs.

DO tell the patient never to stop one of the slow-acting anti-rheumatic drugs once they have worked, unless there are complications.

DO change to another drug if the appropriate duration of therapy has been tried and only a mild effect has been gained.

DON'T stop such drugs because of a complication without a definite plan to either restart the drug, move on to another drug, or refer to a rheumatologist.

Case scenarios

There are many possible scenarios which may be considered regarding the management of rheumatoid arthritis, and with each there may be differing opinions among rheumatologists. The scenarios below are commonly encountered, and the recommendations made are consistent with the current practices of many rheumatologists.

1. A 34-year-old is diagnosed with new-onset rheumatoid arthritis.

Start therapy with:
(a) a visit with a physiotherapist,
(b) a visit with an occupational therapist, and
(c) a check to see if arch supports are needed.

Prescribe NSAID in recommended doses and consider misoprostol cyto-protection. (Some prefer to use lower toxicity NSAIDs, such as trilisate or nabumetone, or to try NSAIDs in lower than recommended doses to see if benefit is still obtained.)

Consider local corticosteroid injections for temporary benefit of involved joints or sites of tendinitis.

Start a slow-acting anti-rheumatic drug at the same time. Any is acceptable, as long as one has checked for contra-indications, and the patient understands what is involved in using these agents (like the need to monitor for complications, to receive injections, etc.). Sulfasalazine and anti-malarial drugs are considered by some rheumatologists to be best for milder disease, and the remainder for more active disease, but there is wide variation in their usage. (Data on minocycline suggests it may also be useful for mild disease.)

American rheumatologists often choose to use low-dose prednisone (prednisolone) in moderate to severe disease, citing the possible need for physiologic replacement, and recent evidence about the effect of corticosteroids on joint erosions. Their use remains controversial to many, however.

Some rheumatologists use systemic corticosteroids to bridge the waiting period for the slow-acting anti-rheumatic drugs. Regimens include methylprednisolone 125 mg IV qd × 3, or 120 mg IM monthly for 6 months. Many rheumatologists, however, rarely resort to parenteral or oral systemic corticosteroids, and yet are successful in treating their patients.

Remind the patient that the slow-acting anti-rheumatic drug is the key to long term therapy, and that they are advised to continue this therapy indefinitely. Remind the patient that they will have to be patient, since slow-acting anti-rheumatic drugs take time to work, and it is hoped that the NSAID, local corticosteroid injections, and advice of the therapists will help in the meantime.

Have some method of objectively documenting the patient's disease activity by counting the number of and location of joint involvement, laboratory measures of activity, etc., as one will need to review the patient and be able to know if improvement has taken place. The patient's input is also, of course, needed.

2. *The same patient as above has been started on gold injections 50 mg weekly for 20 weeks, with a monitoring regimen used. They return at 12 weeks with some improvement.*

If the patient is coping and understands that more time is needed for gold to have its full benefit (at least 20 weekly injections), persist with current therapy.

If the patient has had no improvement at all, most rheumatologists would still advise the patient to persist. One should document objectively the current activity and compare it with the initial assessment (thus the value of having some objective markers at the start of therapy), and should ensure that the complaints the patient has are related to synovitis and not to:
(a) carpal tunnel syndrome,
(b) fibromyalgia (diffuse pains and little or no evidence of synovitis, which means the therapy for RA is working, and a secondary problem of chronic pain is evolving), or
(c) secondary osteoarthritis (see case later).

Also ensure that the patient is receiving the highest recommended and tolerable dose of an NSAID.

3. *The same patient above has no synovitis after 20 weeks of therapy.*

Increase the injection interval to every 2 weeks for 3 months and then reassess. If the patient worsens, examine them to see that it is increased synovitis that is the cause of their symptoms. Patients can have pain for reasons other than active synovitis (i.e. carpal tunnel syndrome, tendinitis/bursitis, or arch collapse).

If they actually have active synovitis, return to weekly injections of gold for another month at least before trying to reduce injection frequency again.

4. *A patient is to be started on gold by injection. After their first injection they develop flushing, pre-syncope, and myalgias and arthralgias.*

If this adverse effect was particularly distressing or serious (patient collapsed) change to an alternate injection preparation. If the patient is willing, a smaller dose can be given (if 50 mg was being used) and the patient monitored in the office to see if the same effects occur.

If the problem persists, use another slow-acting anti-rheumatic drug.

5. *A patient has been on gold therapy (or methotrexate) for a few weeks and routine monitoring of cell counts shows a WBC count of 3.7 × 10⁹/l (normal = 4.0–11.0).*

The options include:

(a) Continue with current therapy as most patients will persist in having a stable white cell count at that level and never develop more significant cytopenia.

(b) Continue with current therapy, but reduce the dose. This can be done if the patient has been responding to the current regimen and if they continue to respond to the lower dose.

(c) Stop the drug until cell counts become normal again (often requires only 1–4 weeks). Do not, however, stop the drug without a plan either to restart it when the cytopenia has resolved or to change to another drug. Leaving a patient with rheumatoid arthritis indefinitely to see if their arthritis will come back is unwise. It will come back, sooner or later.

If the patient is on methotrexate, some would prescribe folic acid 1 mg qd for a few days over the time when the methotrexate is received, to try to reduce marrow suppression, or folinic acid 2.5–5.0 mg the day after methotrexate is received.

6. *A patient is on gold therapy and has protein detected on urine dipstick.*

Collect a 24–hour sample for protein and creatinine clearance.

If the level is less than 0.5 g/24 h, continue therapy and monitoring. If it is more, then stop either the NSAID (if the patient is on one), or the gold or both temporarily. Recheck 24 h urine again in a week. If it persists to be > 0.5 g/24 h, then continue to hold gold for a few more weeks if needed. The gold cannot be held indefinitely, however, since the patient will worsen if proteinuria persists, change to another drug. Gold-induced proteinuria usually resolves within a month. If it does not, a review by a nephrologist is worthwhile. Some cases require systemic corticosteroid therapy, and it would be worthwhile to justify such therapy with a renal biopsy confirming the diagnosis. It would also be an opportunity to look for other causes of proteinuria (diabetes, hypertension, other drugs, etc.).

7. *A 54-year-old man has been on methotrexate 15 mg by injection weekly for 8 weeks, and has failed to improve significantly.*

Compare the patient's condition objectively with that when his therapy was started. Check to see that the patient actually has synovitis as the cause of their symptoms.

Offer temporary relief by ensuring that the patient is receiving the highest tolerable, recommended dose of an NSAID, using local corticosteroid injections at involved sites, consider parenteral corticosteroids as discussed above, and if needed, hospitalization and physiotherapy.

One could then increase the dose of methotrexate by 2.5 to 5.0 mg (rheumatologists vary according to how often and how much they will adjust the methotrexate dose). If higher doses cause gastrointestinal symptoms, one could give folic acid 1 mg qd for the few days overlapping the time when the methotrexate is received or folinic acid 2.5–5.0 mg the day after methotrexate is received .

This, together with temporary relief, may be sufficient and should work over the next 4–8 weeks. If not, consider increasing the dose by another 2.5–5.0 mg until the dose is effective (go up to as much as 35 mg if needed, but get advice from a rheumatologist above a dose of 20 mg/week) or becomes intolerable (even when the patient is on folic or folinic acid). Alternatively, one could add sulfasulazine or change to another drug altogether. Consider involving a rheumatologist at this time.

8. A 45-year-old woman has been on sulfasalazine 1.0 g po bid, and has done well except for increasing knee pain.

When one examines the patient, one will find no evidence of active synovitis anywhere except small effusions in both knees. Further examination reveals decreased knee range of motion, crepitus, and ligament laxity. This patient has secondary osteoarthritis of the knees and will not likely benefit from any change in slow-acting anti-rheumatic drug or increase in its dose.

The treatment of her osteoarthritis involves perhaps determining if she needs arch supports, orthotic knee supports, a cane, corticosteroid injection, and depending on the severity of the patient's symptoms, and the response to these measures, eventual surgery. (See section on osteoarthritis, page 92).

9. A 55-year-old woman on penicillamine therapy has been doing poorly, with pain in the shoulders, wrists, knees, and toes. Her former physician had taken her off gold therapy which was initially beneficial, but now these symptoms have occurred, and penicillamine was started 4 months ago with little benefit.

One might be tempted to change the penicillamine dose, or change to another drug. Instead one decides to ask the patient about symptoms of carpal tunnel syndrome, and examines her shoulders, hands, knees, and feet. One finds that she actually has bilateral shoulder tendinitis, carpal tunnel syndrome, secondary osteoarthritis of both knees, and arch collapse. (See sections on osteoarthritis, the painful shoulder, and the painful foot or ankle for treatment recommendations for these disorders pages 92, 42 and 83 respectively.)

The rheumatoid arthritis is actually controlled, and these symptoms are not a reflection of a need to change the slow-acting anti-rheumatic drug. This emphasizes the importance of carefully evaluating the cause of pain in a patient with rheumatoid arthritis. Tendinitis, arch collapse, osteoarthritis, and neuropathy are common in rheumatoid arthritis and do not require any changes in slow-acting anti-rheumatic drug therapy.

10. *A patient with rheumatoid arthritis is to be started on gold therapy. A complete cell count is carried out.*

(a) Hgb	10.1 g/l (normal = 13.0–17.0)
(b) WBC	10.9×10^9/l (normal = 4.5–11.0)
(c) Differential	Slight increase in lymphocytes
(d) Platelets	420×10^9/l (normal = 130–400)
(e) Mean cell volume	79 fl (normal = 83–97)

You are concerned about possible gastrointestinal blood loss because the patient has a microcytic anemia.

Actually, this phenomenon is common in rheumatoid arthritis, particularly when the disease is very active. Most rheumatologists do not pursue any further investigations at this stage, but will wait until disease activity is reduced, and see if there is an improvement in the hemoglobin. A serum ferritin below 100 μg/l is, however, suggestive of iron deficiency (because the chronic inflammatory state normally elevates it well above this).

Investigations are usually only carried out further if the patient gives a history of gastrointestinal blood loss, or if the anemia is profound and mean cell volume is very low (although even in these cases, the cause will sometimes be the disease activity, and investigations will be negative).

11. *A patient on an antimalarial drug develops a sudden flare in his right knee, with swelling, pain, and restriction of movement.*

You notice that there is no other joint involvement.

This patient has septic arthritis until proven otherwise. Joint aspiration for Gram stain and culture, and for crystals is required.

12. *A patient has just been started on methotrexate and is being monitored with weekly CBC. The patient is found to have a WBC of 0.2×10^9/l. (normal = 4.5–11.0).*

Get this patient into hospital, stop the methotrexate, and give IV folinic acid (get the help of a hematologist or rheumatologist).

If the patient has fever, broad spectrum antibiotic coverage for Gram-negative organisms is necessary after careful examination for possible site of infection, including throat swabs, blood and urine cultures, and chest X-ray.

Appendix 1

Physiotherapy exercises

The exercises described in this appendix are written for the patient's instruction. There are many different approaches to writing a 'prescription' of exercises. In general, acute forms of tendinitis or bursitis will often respond to medical therapy alone (especially corticosteroid injections) but chronic tendinitis on the other hand, especially with muscular atrophy, will often not respond to medical therapy alone, so exercises are required. Keep the exercise prescription simple, and encourage the patient to do them independently, at home. Ask them to return in a few days or a week to make sure the exercises are being done properly. If you are going to involve a physiotherapist, two visits only are needed, one to teach the exercises, and one to check that the patient is doing them properly. The exercises should be done until the patient is asymptomatic and, in the case of muscle atrophy, until the atrophy is resolved. Exercise prescriptions for various disorders are described below with the numbered exercises following.

THE SHOULDER

For shoulder tendinitis, bursitis, or minor rotator cuff tears with symptoms for less than 2 months

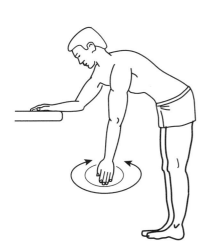

Use medical therapy with Exercise 1. This is often sufficient. If there is evidence of supraspinatus atrophy, add Exercise 10a. If this strengthening exercise is added Exercise 1 should immediatelyt precede and follow it to adequately stretch the muscles.

For shoulder tendinitis, bursitis, or significant rotator cuff tears with symptoms for more than 2 months
Medical therapy is less useful, and one should definitely use Exercises 1, along with 10a, 10b and 10c. Of the latter, 10a is the most important, so if you are trying to keep the exercise prescription simple for the patient, you may choose Exercise 1 and 10a alone.

Exercise 1

For adhesive capsulitis (frozen shoulder)
In addition to medical therapy, prescribe at least some of the Exercises 1, 2 (or 3 or 6), 4, 5, 7, 8 (or 9). When the range of motion is nearly normal with these mobilization exercises, add the strengthening Exercises 10a, 10b, and 10c, gradually reducing the mobilization exercises and doing more of the strengthening exercises.

For chronic shoulder arthritis
In addition to medical therapy, emphasize the strengthening Exercises 10a, 10b, and 10c.

Swinging arms in circles (Exercise 1)
Pendulum exercises to maintain mobility can be done seated or standing. Lean forward and to the side of the painful shoulder. Support yourself with the good arm if needed. With your affected arm relaxed and hanging, swing your arm to make small circles of motion (say 30 cm diameter) for about 1 min, alternating clockwise and counter-clockwise. Hold a weight (2.25 kg) in your hand to increase the stretch. Do this exercise several times a day, and whenever the shoulder is painful. If you are doing any strengthening exercises, this stretching exercise should be done before and after those exercises.

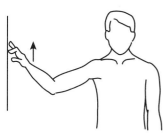

Exercise 2

Fingers climb up wall (Exercise 2)
In this exercise, you are seated or standing about 30–60 cm from a wall, with your affected shoulder closest to the wall, so that the fingers can easily reach the wall without having to move the arm too far away from the body. Reach out to the wall, and crawl upwards with your fingers gripping along it, using the fingers to help keep the arm up. Slowly increase the distance up the wall, always with your arm directly out to the side, and with your trunk always upright. The point at which pain is felt should be noted. Hold the arm there for 10 sec, then crawl back down the wall slowly being sure not to let the arm fall. Each time try to reach a little higher up the wall, but do not cheat by bending your trunk rather than moving your shoulder to get your arm up higher. Do 10 repetitions, twice daily.

If this exercise is too painful, you may find it easier to do it facing the wall, and letting the fingers climb up the wall. When this can be accomplished without difficulty, the above exercise can then be tried.

Assisted shoulder stretch to side (Left arm is used to stretch right shoulder) (Exercise 3)
An alternative to the finger-climbing method of stretching is to place the end of a stick or broom handle in the palm of your affected side. Either seated or standing, you can grasp the other end of the stick or broom with the good arm,

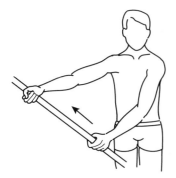

and push your affected arm sideways by using the good arm to push in that direction. Your affected arm is then pushed by the good arm to the highest tolerable height, held there for 10 sec, then slowly lowered. Do 10 repetitions, twice daily.

Exercise 3

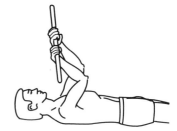

Overhead shoulder stretch (Exercise 4)
Grasp the ends of the stick in front of your body, **Exercise 4**
and then using your good arm to do the work,
slowly lift the stick horizontally up and over your head to be placed in behind your neck, or merely above your head. Hold for 10 sec, and bring both arms slowly back to the starting position. Do 10 repetitions, twice daily.

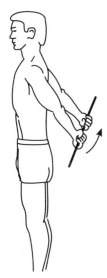

Behind-the-back stretch (Exercise 5)
Hold the stick behind your body and grasp with both hands, raise your arms backwards, letting your good arm do the work, thus extending your shoulder. Hold for 10 sec, and bring both arms slowly back to the starting position. Do 10 repetitions, twice daily.

One arm pulls the other one up (Exercise 6)
Finally, another mobility exercise can be done with a pulley system. Place a rope over a door handle, for instance, which acts as the pulley, and sit on the

Exercise 5

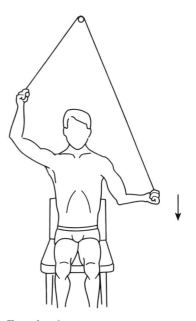

floor. Sit with your head closest to the pulley, and your feet away from it. Grasp the ends of the rope in each hand, with the rope over the pulley. Hold your arms straight out to the sides. Use your good arm to pull on the rope and this will automatically elevate your

Exercise 6

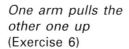

Physiotherapy exercises

affected arm. Keep the arms relatively straight. Do this slowly until a full range of motion is achieved or discomfort is felt. Hold the arm at that position for 10 sec, then slowly lower it to the original position. Do 10 repetitions, twice daily.

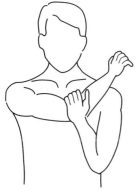

Across-body shoulder stretch (Exercise 7)

While standing, use your good arm to grasp the wrist of your affected arm. Pull your affected arm slowly across the front of the body as far as is comfortable, and hold for 10 sec, then slowly release. Next, grasp your affected arm again, but this time from behind the back, and attempt to pull the arm across the back of the body as far as comfortable and hold for 10 sec. One can alternate these two exercises or do one 10 times, before proceeding to the other. Do 10 repetitions, twice daily.

Exercise 7

Stretching shoulder against wall (Exercise 8)

While standing, place the affected arm on a wall near a corner or doorway. With the forearm held against the wall, step forward past the corner or through the doorway to stretch the shoulder as much as comfortable, then hold for a few seconds. Return to the resting position slowly. Do 10 repetitions, twice daily.

Stretching shoulder against table (Exercise 9)

While kneeling or standing, place the affected arm on a flat surface, with the table or other surface at the side of the body, and at a lower level than the shoulder. Lower the body slowly and gently to as low as comfortable, then hold for a few seconds. Slowly return to the resting position. Do 10 repetitions, twice daily.

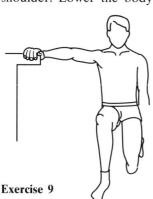

Exercise 8

Exercise 9

Strengthening exercises for the shoulder (Exercise 10)

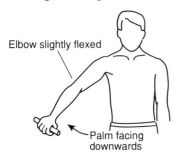

Elbow slightly flexed

Palm facing downwards

Starting with your hands in front of your thighs, raise them slowly out towards the side until they are at about 45° from your body, with palms facing down. Hold for 5 sec, then slowly lower them to the starting position in front of your thighs. Keep the elbow slightly bent during the movement. When this can be done with 10 repetitions, twice daily, then add a small weight (0.5–2.5 kg) in each hand. Increase the weight by 1–2 kg when you can do 10 repetitions, twice daily. Continue until you have achieved the exercise with a weight of 5–7 kg in each hand. (*Exercise 10a*)

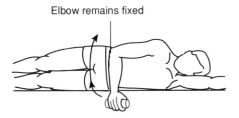

Elbow remains fixed

Exercise 10b1

Lie on your side with the affected shoulder up, your arm held against the side of your trunk and your elbow flexed to 90°. Pick up a weight from the floor, and while keeping your elbow against the trunk, lift the weight up slowly to as far as is comfortable. Then lower it slowly (*Exercise 10b1*).

This exercise can be done in a chair with an elastic cord tied to a fixed site. With your elbow bent, and keeping the upper arm against your side, pull on the cord, moving across your body, and hold for 5 sec. Then release slowly (*Exercise 10b2*).

Lie on your back or side with your affected arm held close to your side and elbow bent 90°. Pick up a weight on the floor and raise it across the body by rotating the arm, keeping your elbow pressed against the floor and against your body. (*Exercise 10c1*).

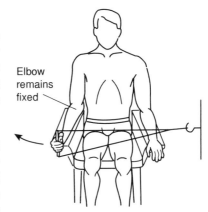

Elbow remains fixed

Exercise 10b2

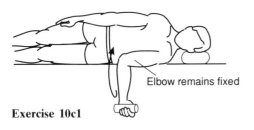

Elbow remains fixed

Exercise 10c1

This exercise can be done in a chair with an elastic cord tied to a fixed site. With your elbow bent, and keeping your upper arm against your side, pull on the cord, moving away from your body, and hold for 5 sec. Then release slowly (*Exercise 10c2*).

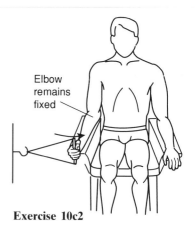

Elbow remains fixed

Exercise 10c2

TENNIS ELBOW, GOLFER'S ELBOW, AND HAND TENDINITIS

Exercise prescriptions for various disorders are described below with the numbered exercises following.

For tennis elbow with symptoms of less than 2 months
Use medical therapy with Exercise 11a. This is often sufficient. If the patient is having recurrences due to overuse, add the strengthening Exercise 11b.

The strengthening exercise should only begin, however, when the extensors are flexible enough that the wrist can be flexed at 90° with the elbow straight, producing only mild discomfort. Use of strengthening exercises without achieving flexibility only increases extensor muscle tightness further.

For tennis elbow with symptoms of more than 2 months
Medical therapy is less useful, and one should definitely prescribe Exercise 11a followed by 11b when flexibility is achieved.

For golfer's elbow with symptoms of less than 2 months
Use Exercise 12a, adding 12b if patient is having recurrences. The strengthening exercise should only begin, however, when the extensors are flexible enough that the wrist can be flexed to 90° with the elbow straight, producing only mild discomfort. Use of strengthening exercises without achieving flexibility only increases extensor muscle tightness further.

For golfer's elbow with symptoms of more than 2 months
Medical therapy is less useful, and one should definitely prescribe Exercise 12a followed by 12b when flexibility is achieved.

For hand tendinitis
Often corticosteroid injection therapy is sufficient, but an approach similar to that for tennis or golfer's elbow could be used, depending on whether it is extensor or flexor hand tendinitis.

Elbow stretching exercises

The muscles that are on the inner surface of your forearm which act to make a fist and curl the fist towards you are called the flexors. The muscles on the outer surface of your forearm are called the extensors. Do 10 repetitions of each exercise, and do the sequence of exercises twice daily.

Stretching forearm extensors (Exercise 11a)
Stand near a wall, with your affected arm closest to the wall. Place the back of your hand flat against the wall at waist height, the fingers pointing down. Slowly raise the hand up along the wall. This will cause the wrist to bend and stretch the muscles. Raise the hand up as high as comfortable (or until there is a pulling sensation at the elbow), and hold there for 10 sec, then lower it slowly.

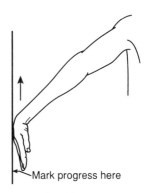

Mark progress here

Exercise 11a

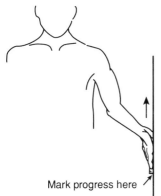

Stretching forearm flexors (Exercise 11b)
For stretching the flexors, stand near a wall, with your affected arm closest to the wall and thumb backward. Place the palm of your hand flat against the wall at waist height, with your fingers pointing down. Slowly raise your hand up along the wall. This will cause the wrist to bend and stretch the muscles. Raise your hand up as high as comfortable (or until there is a pulling sensation at the elbow), and hold there for 10 sec, then lower slowly.

Mark progress here

Exercise 11b

Elbow strengthening exercises

For strengthening, use a light weight (0.5–2.5 kg) initially. Do 5–10 repetitions of each exercise twice daily. Increase weight by 1.0–2.0 kg when you can easily do 10 repetitions, twice daily, and continue until you have achieved the exercise with a weight of 5–7 kg.

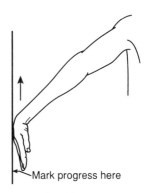

Exercise 12a

Strengthening forearm extensors (Exercise 12a)
Lay your affected forearm on a flat surface such as a table with your hand hanging loosely off the end, and palm facing down. Grasp the weight in your hand and slowly raise the weight by bending (extending) the wrist only. Hold this for 5 sec and slowly lower to the resting position.

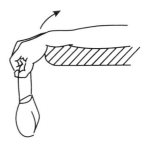

Strengthening forearm flexors (Exercise 12b)
Use the same arm position as above, but this time with your palm facing upward. Grasp the weight and slowly raise it by bending (flexing) the wrist only. Hold the weight for 5 sec and slowly lower.

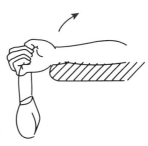

Exercise 12b

PATELLAR BURSITIS, PATELLOFEMORAL SYNDROME, AND KNEE ARTHRITIS

Strengthening of the quadriceps muscles can be helpful in all of these conditions and these exercises are the most commonly recommended for therapy.

Quadriceps exercise (Exercise 13)

There are many different methods of doing this exercise. One method is to sit on a chair or another surface with the thighs completely supported. Place your feet on a rest so that your knees are slightly or halfway flexed. Place a pillow between your knees and squeeze it. Then lift your feet together, straightening your knees and holding straight for 10 sec. Repeat 10 times. When this can be done easily add a small weight (2 kg) to each ankle and again to 10 repetitions, holding each one for 10 sec. Continue to increase the weight by 2 kg as your strength increases, until you have about 7–10 kg on each ankle.

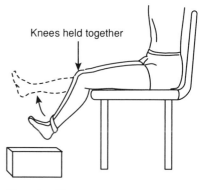

Knees held together

Exercise 13

ANKLE TENDINITIS AND CALF MUSCLE STRAINS

These exercises can be used for calf strains, Achilles tendinitis, and other forms of tendinitis about the ankle. Stretching is the chief aim.

Exercises for lower leg disorders

For tendinitis of the ankle, or for calf muscle strains, these exercises can be helpful, not only for treatment but also for warm-up and cool-down exercises before and after activities.

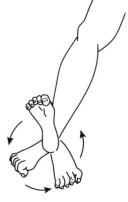

Exercise 14

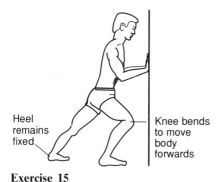

Heel remains fixed

Knee bends to move body forwards

Exercise 15

Ankle rotation (Exercise 14)

Rest your legs on a stool or chair with the foot hanging free from support. Then curl your toes and while keeping them curled, make 10–30 rotations of the ankle clockwise, then counterclockwise twice a day.

Calf stretch (Exercise 15)

Stand facing a wall (30–60 cm away), and place your palms firmly along the wall at shoulder height. Step with one leg to support your body as you lean forward to bring your head towards the wall, keeping your heels on the floor, until there is stretching in the back of the calf. Hold this for 30 sec. Then switch legs. If the exercise is easy, slide the leg being stretched back 18–20 cm and try stretching again. Repeat 5–10 times on each leg, and the exercise twice daily.

Calf and hamstring stretch (Exercise 16)

This exercise can be used to stretch both the hamstring (back of the thigh) muscles and the calf muscles. Lie on your back and place a rope behind the ball of your foot, grasping one end of the rope in each hand. Raise your leg up to near vertical, and pull on the rope. This will cause a stretching sensation of the calf and hamstring muscles. Hold this for 30 sec, repeat stretch 5–10 times, and twice daily.

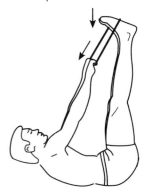

Foot pulled into stretch

Exercise 16

Alternative method for calf stretch (Exercise 17)

This exercise can be used to stretch and strengthen the calf muscles. Stand on a step with the balls of your foot on the step, and the heel and remainder of the foot hanging free, level with the step. Hold on to the railing or other support, and slowly lower your heels, stretching the calves, and feeling a pulling sensation there. Hold for 30 sec, and then raise yourself back up for a few seconds, then repeat the stretching 5–10 times, and the exercise twice daily. If raising the heels back is too difficult, climb down from the step, and then return to the starting position, and lower yourself again.

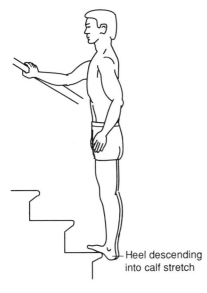

Heel descending into calf stretch

Exercise 17

MECHANICAL BACK PAIN

A few of the exercises are described below. They are not done in disc protrusion with nerve impingement, until the pain is considerably improved. For more information see *The Back Doctor* (see further reading, page 232). In general, one selects the exercises based on the pattern of mechanical back pain (see topic The Painful Back, page 146). For pattern 1 or 3 back pain, use posture advice (Exercises 21a, b and c). For pattern 2 back pain, use Exercises 18 and 19. For pattern 4 back pain, use Exercises 18, 19, 20 and hamstring stretches of any type.

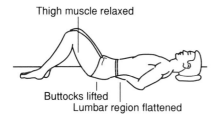

Thigh muscle relaxed

Buttocks lifted
Lumbar region flattened

Exercise 18

Pelvic tilt (Exercise 18)

The pelvic tilt can be done lying on your back, with your knees bent. The abdominal muscles are used to flatten the lumbar region (low region) of the back, and to raise the buttocks slightly. The buttocks should not be raised, however, by pushing with your feet. You may find this exercise easier to do if you place one hand behind your back, and feel your hand being pressed on by your lower back when the pelvic tilt is done properly. Hold the pelvic tilt for 5–10 sec and repeat five times. Increase the number of repetitions as you get stronger. Another way to do the pelvic tilt is to stand with your back against the wall with heels, buttocks, and shoulders touching the wall. Now attempt to place the low back flat against the wall. A pelvic tilt is required to do this.

Pelvic tilt and abdominal crunch (Exercise 19)

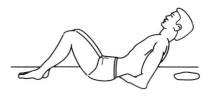

Exercise 19

Lying on your back with knees bent, use the abdominal muscles to flatten the back and lift the shoulders off the floor. Do not pull with the head and neck to get the upper body off the floor. The movement must come from the abdomen. This exercise will also result in the lumbar region of the back becoming flat. Hold the position for 5–10 sec and repeat five times, again increasing the number of repetitions as you get stronger. If you have a proven pinched nerve, this exercise may be painful, and should be avoided if it causes pain. You can combine this exercise with the pelvic tilt, attempting to draw in the knees toward the chest without using the arms. This is essentially curling your body. Hold this position for 5 sec and repeat five times.

Back stretch (Exercise 20)

Lying on your back, grasp behind your knees with both hands, and pull the knees towards the chest. This is a good stretch to do early in attacks of back pain.

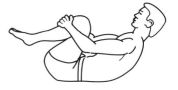

Exercise 20

Methods to correct poor posture (Exercise 21)

Postural changes include consciously holding your shoulders back, and avoiding the slouching posture whenever you can. To make it easier to maintain good posture without having to think about it, you should always sit with

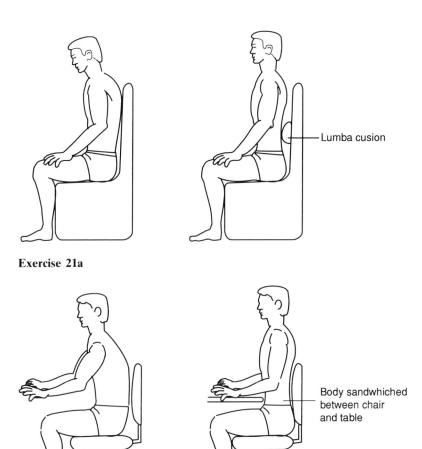

Exercise 21a

Lumba cusion

Body sandwhiched between chair and table

Exercise 21b

a small cushion along your lower back (lumbar region). This forces you to assume a more upright posture (*Exercise 21a*). In the same sense, whenever you are sitting at a table or desk, you should be seated with your back against the chair, and the chair pulled forward so that your abdomen reaches the table or desk (*Exercise 21b*). This also improves your posture.

The other thing you can try if you have a slouched posture, with shoulders curling forward, is to do a daily exercise in which you lie on your abdomen,

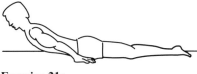

Exercise 21c

and without the aid of the arms lift the head and shoulders from the floor, arching your back (*Exercise 21c*). This position can be held for 10 sec, and then repeated several times, gradually increasing the number of repetitions. If your

spine has become used to having a poor posture, you may find this painful
initially. It is painful because your spine has become stiff after months or years
of poor posture. The pain of doing this exercise is to be expected, and will go
away as you continue to stretch the spine into a normal posture.

THE NECK

Neck stretches

The neck stretch below is useful for whiplash, and any neck pain with tender
or tight neck muscles, as long as the patient understands that this stretch is
initially painful, but that this pain is due to simply stretching sore muscles.
While the patient has neck pain, it is also very important that they use the
posture advice above for mechanical back pain (Exercises 21a and 21b), as
improvement in the lumbar spine posture improves the cervical spine posture.
Patients with neck pain tend to ease their pain by keeping their neck forward,
but this only promotes further muscle tightness. This advice alone will manage
most neck pain, and other exercises are not needed.

Front-to-back neck stretch
(Exercise 22)

Looking straight ahead without
your head tilted up or down, pull
your chin inward (to make a
'double chin') so as to flatten the
curve of your neck. You will find
this causes pain along the muscles
of the neck and upper back. It
should. This means you are doing
the exercise properly and are

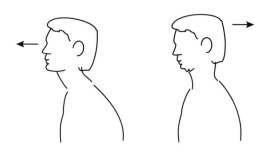

Exercise 22

stretching tight neck muscles. As you continue the exercise, you will remove
the tightness from these muscles, and the exercise eventually becomes painless.

Hold the stretch for 5 sec, and then stretch your neck out forwards. Repeat
this process ten times, frequently throughout the day, and whenever your neck
is particularly painful.

Appendix 2

Soft-tissue inflammatory disorders (including shoulder arthritis)

Disorder	History	Examination
Impingement syndrome (Rotator cuff tendinitis)	Pain over anterolateral shoulder Pain when lying on that shoulder	Painful arc of abduction 60–120° Positive impingement signs Tenderness over greater tuberosity
Calcific tendinitis	Very sudden onset As above	As above X-ray shows calcification
Biceps tendinitis	Pain anteriorly Pain when carrying objects	Pain with resisted shoulder flexion Pain over biceps tendon between greater and lesser tuberosities
Adhesive capsulitis	Pain deep and anterior Marked stiffness	Restriction of active and passive movement in all directions Prominent restriction of external rotation
Acromioclavicular arthritis	Pain over anterolateral shoulder	Painful arc of abduction from 90–180° Tender over joint
Sternoclavicular arthritis	Pain over clavicle Painful during most movements	Painful arc of abduction 90-180° Tender over joint
Glenohumeral arthritis	Pain over anterolateral shoulder	Painful arc of abduction 90–180° Painful internal rotation Restriction of active and passive internal rotation
Tennis elbow	Pain over lateral elbow, forearm Pain with gripping activities	Painful resisted wrist extension Painful when asked to grip Pain lessened when muscles splinted Tender over lateral humeral epicondyle

Disorder	History	Examination
Golfer's elbow	Pain over medial elbow, forearm Pain with gripping activities	Painful resisted wrist flexion Painful when asked to grip Tender over medial humeral epicondyle
Olecranon bursitis	Painful swelling at elbow tip Possibly history of gout	Obvious swelling over olecranon
De Quervain's tendinitis	Pain over radial aspect of wrist, thumb Pain with gripping 'handle of kettle and lifting'	Finklestein's sign Tender over tendon
Hand or foot tendinitis	Pain over wrist, ankle, or small joints	May have swelling and look like arthritis, but passive range of movement is better than active
Trochanteric bursitis	Pain over lateral upper thigh 'Hip pain, Doc' Pain worse when lying on side and at night	Normal hip range of movement Tender right over trochanter
Patellar tendinitis	Pain over anterior knee Pain with jumping	Pain with resisted knee extension Tenderness at inferior patella
Pre-patellar bursitis	Pain over anterior knee Pain worse with kneeling	Swelling and tender over inferior patella
Infra-patellar bursitis	Pain over anterior knee Pain worse with kneeling	Swelling under patellar tendon Tender under patellar tendon
Anserine bursitis	Pain over medial knee Pain on kneeling	Normal knee range of movement Tender over anserine bursa
Plantar fasciitis	Pain over heel and sole of foot Worse when walking, especially in a.m.	Tender over heel
Plantar arch collapse	Pain under toes, dorsum of foot Pain in ankle Pain over anterior tibia	No swelling Arch collapse
Morton's neuroma	Pain over toes, sometimes shooting	Normal MTP range of movement Pain on compression between toes, not over actual MTP joints

Appendix 3

Joint aspiration and injection techniques

Joint aspiration, corticosteroid injections, and more recently, viscosupplement injections for osteoarthritis are essential skills in dealing with rheumatic diseases. The techniques are best learnt by hands-on teaching sessions, as even most 'injection manuals' cannot fully convey the skills needed. The discussion below will be limited to concepts to be considered when using such techniques, and how to best use them to the patient's benefit.

General comments

1. It is important to explain to the patient why the procedure is indicated, what will be done, the risks, benefits, and alternatives. One should also ask about allergy to local anesthetics or corticosteroid preparations, and about the use of anticoagulants or existence of a known bleeding diasthesis. The adverse effects, which may include allergic reaction, infection (rare), and skin hypo- or hyperpigmentation at the injection site should be explained. (The last is avoided by not permitting any subcutaneous injection of the corticosteroid.)

2. Sterile technique varies greatly among clinicians. Some use simply an alcohol or iodinated swab at the aspiration site, while others use a broader surface of disinfection, sterile drapes, and sterile gloves. (Most tend to use the less stringent techniques.) Infection following aspiration or injection is a rare event, in any case. A more careful sterile technique may instead be most important when one is suspicious of septic arthritis or bursitis, and does not want to introduce bacteria from the skin or other sources to contaminate the sample. Local infection of skin or periarticular tissues is a contraindication to needle puncture into the joint (unless septic arthritis is suspected) since one may introduce infection.

3. The use of local anesthesia prior to aspirations or injection is common. If one is using a small gauge needle, say 21–25 gauge, and the procedure is relatively quickly completed, the needle puncture of anesthesia may be just as uncomfortable to the patient as the procedure itself. In such cases, anesthesia may have little benefit for the patient. If using a larger gauge needle (often done when one is suspecting a viscous fluid return, as in septic arthritis), if the area is quite tender, or if the procedure may prove more difficult, local anaesthesia with a small gauge needle (25 gauge) may be

quite useful. If a small joint of the hand or foot is to be aspirated, and it is quite tender, a 'ring' block can be used to anesthetize the entire digit. One should be aware that lidocaine injection into the joint or bursal fluid in significant amounts (probably more than 10 ml of a 2% lidocaine solution) may result in bacterial culture inhibition and misleading results. An alternative to lidocaine anesthesia is chloroethane spray.

4. Obtain a sufficient sample for each test desired. A heparinized, or EDTA-containing tube prevents clotting of the sample (important for cell counts, crystal analysis). Sterile tubes should be used for Gram stain and culture. If the return in the needle is a small amount of fluid or only enough to fill the needle, this can be sent for culture by depositing the entire needle (capped: if the cap is still sterile) and syringe to the microbiology lab (forewarning them of the needle). Alternatively, one may aspirate culture broth into the needle and syringe and inject the mixture back into the culture medium under sterile technique (which is what the laboratory will do with small samples).

5. Use 2.5–3.25 cm (1–1½ inches) needles for carpal tunnel, glenohumeral joint, knee joint, ankle joint, bursal, biceps tendon sheath, and plantar fascia injections. Use 1.5 cm or 1.25 cm (½–⅝ inch) for small joints, and longer (spinal type) needles for femoral trochanteric bursa injections.

6. Infections tend to produce a viscous, purulent, sometimes bloody effusion, whereas other inflammatory conditions tend to produce decreased viscosity form the normal synovial fluid (especially rheumatoid arthritis). See *Table 1*.

    The synovial fluid characteristics of various forms of arthritis are listed in *Table 2*.

7. Crystals (sodium urate, calcium pyrophosphate) should be examined for the same day since many disappear in the first 12–24 h. Sodium urate crystals (seen in gout) are needle shaped, about as long as the diameter of a white cell, negatively birefringent, and often intracellular. Calcium pyrophosphate crystals (pseudogout) are shorter, rhomboid (and sometimes a mixture of needle-shaped, rhomboid, and indistinct forms) positively birefringent, seldom intracellular. The absence of crystals does not exclude crystal arthropathy, and one may have to repeat the aspiration on the next event to make a diagnosis.

8. When injecting or aspirating at sites of active synovitis, the simplest approach is to insert the needle at the site of maximal swelling, since this represents distension of the joint capsule which is often distended well beyond the bony confines of the joint. The aim is not to insert the needle tip between the bones of the joint, but rather through the joint capsule, being intimately lined by the synovium. In joints with much less swelling it is important to know the landmarks that will allow one to guide the needle through the joint capsule.

Table 1 Causes of bloody effusion

Septic arthritis
Trauma
Crystal arthritis
Avascular necrosis
Bleeding diasthesis
Villonodular synovioma

Table 2 Synovial fluid characteristics in arthritis

Disease	WBC (mm^{-3})	Predominant cell type	Glucose	Viscosity	Appearance
Osteoarthritis	< 3000	Monocyte	Normal	Normal	Clear, amber
Trauma	< 3000	Monocyte	Normal	Normal/low	Clear, amber, or bloody
Rheumatoid arthritis, crystal arthopathy,or seronegative spondylo-arthropathy	3000–50000	Neutrophils, monocytes	Normal/low	Low	Cloudy, yellow
Infection	>30 000	Neutrophil	Low	Variable	Purulent or bloody

Corticosteroid injections

1.   There are many corticosteroid preparations available for injection, some with pre-mixed local anesthetic. (*Table 3*). Further details about how to use of each are available in drug monographs. Some clinicians inject lidocaine 0.5% (2 ml), 1.0% (1 ml), or 2% (0.5 ml) prior to corticosteroid injection. It is not recommended by the manufacturers that the corticosteroid otherwise be mixed with a possibly incompatible local anesthetic, unless a pre-mixed formulation is provided. If the two drugs are used separately, then use the same needle for each solution by making the puncture, injecting the local anesthetic, and without removing the needle from its location, change to the syringe with corticosteroid, and inject this. Most corticosteroid formulations inject easily through a number 25 or 27 gauge needle, which may be less uncomfortable for the patient.

2.   DO NOT inject corticosteroid into a region unless you are confident that there is no infection. One may have to perform aspiration of a swollen joint, for example, to rule out infection (and to verify the diagnosis), and wait for Gram stain and culture results prior to injection. Other contraindications are listed in *Table 4*.

3.   Many patients will benefit from the injection immediately (from the lidocaine), and within 1–4 days from the corticosteroid. The inflammatory

Table 3 Corticosteroid dosage and type according to site of injection (volume in ml)

Corticosteroid	Most sites	Hand/foot joints Sternoclavicular Acromioclavicular
Methylprednisolone(Depo-Medrol®) 20 mg/ml	2.0–4.0	0.2–0.5
Methylprednisolone(Depo-Medrol®) 40 mg/ml	1.0–2.0	0.1–0.25
Methylprednisolone(Depo-Medrol®) 80 mg/ml	0.5–1.0	0.1
Triamcinolone (Kenalog®) 10 mg/ml	4.0–6.0	0.4–1.0
Triamcinolone (Aristopspan®) 20 mg/ml	2.0–4.0	0.2–0.5
Triamcinolone (Kenalog®) 40 mg/ml	1.0–2.0	0.1–0.25
Betametasone (Celestone Soluspan®) 6 mg/ml	1.0–2.0	0.1–0.25
Dexamethasone (Decadron®, Hexadrol®) 4 mg/ml	1.2–2.4	0.1-0.4
Dexamethasone (Decadron-LA®) 8 mg/ml	0.6–1.2	0.1–0.2
Prednisolone (Hydeltra-TBA®) 20 mg/ml	2.5–5.0	0.25–0.75

condition may worsen or 'flare', however, for the first 1–2 days, possibly as a reaction to the corticosteroid. Persistence of this flare beyond 3 days, however, suggests incorrect diagnosis (i.e. Did the patient have septic arthritis?)

4. Avoid injection into tendons. Having the patient flex and extend the joint may be helpful (if the needle is in the tendon, it will move with flexion and extension).

    It is generally recommended that no more than three injections per year be done within a joint, tendon sheath, or ligaments since there is an increased risk of tendon or ligament rupture with more injections. There may also an increased risk of avascular necrosis and Charcot-like arthropathy.

5. Aspirating fluid prior to injection of a largely swollen joint offers some relief in itself, but also dilutes the injected corticosteroid less. One may aspirate a small amount of joint fluid into the syringe containing the corticosteroid to help confirm appropriate location.

Table 4   Contraindications to local corticosteroid injection

An unstable joint
Avascular necrosis
Bleeding diasthesis
Fracture in joint
Infection within or near injection site
Presence of joint prosthesis
Prior history of tuberculosis[a]
Rotator cuff tear

[a] Cases of reactivation within the joint have been reported. Although one could give prophylactic isoniazid for 6 months when the injection is given, corticosteroid injections are not so essential as to go to that extreme. Find another source of therapy.

Further reading

1. McCarty D J and Koopman W J (1993) *Arthritis and Allied Conditions*. 12th edn. Pennsylvania, Lea and Febiger.
2. Maddison P J, Isenberg D A, Woo P and Glass D N (1993) *Oxford Textbook of Rheumatology*. Oxford, Oxford University Press.
3. Kelley W N, Harris E D, Jr, Ruddy S and Sledge C B (1993) *Textbook of Rheumatology*. 4th edn. Philadelphia, W.B. Saunders Co.
4. Sheon R P, Moskowitz R W and Goldberg V M (1987) *Soft Tissue Rheumatic Pain*. 2nd edn. Philadelphia, Lea and Febiger.
5. Hall H (1980) *The Back Doctor*. Toronto, McClelland-Bantam Inc.

Index

Abortion
and antiphospholipid antibodies, 21
ACE inhibitors, *see* Angiotensin-
converting enzyme inhibitors
Acetaminophen (paracetamol)
analgesic effect compared to NSAIDs,
193
in osteoarthritis, 96, 97
Acetylsalicylic acid, 194
Achilles tendinitis, *see* Tendinitis,
Achilles
AIDS (Acquired immunodeficiency
syndrome)
psoriatic arthritis in, 141
Reiter's syndrome in, 140
Gram-negative septic arthritis in, 114
ACR, *see* American College of
Rheumatology
Acromioclavicular joint, *see* shoulder
Adverse drug effects, *see under specific*
drug names
Algodystrophy, *see* Reflex sympathetic
dystrophy
Allergic vasculitis, *see* Vasculitis, small-
vessel
Allopurinol, 106, 109, 110
Alkaline phosphatase
in metabolic bone disease, 180
Alkylating agents, *see* Chlorambucil,
Cyclophosphamide
American College of Rheumatology
diagnostic criteria
fibromyalgia, 14
giant cell arteritis, 14
rheumatoid arthritis, 12
American Rheumatism Association
diagnostic criteria
rheumatoid arthritis, 12
systemic lupus erythematosus, 12

systemic sclerosis, 13
Aminoglycosides
in septic arthritis, 114
ANA, *see* Antibodies, Antinuclear
Anemia
drug-induced, 201
in rheumatoid arthritis, 120, 122
in systemic lupus erythematosus, 12,
127, 129, 131
Anaesthesia, local
for joint aspiration, 225
for corticosteroid injections, 227
Anaphylactoid purpura, *see* Vasculitis,
small-vessel
ANCA, *see* antineutrophil cytoplasmic
antibodies
Angiitis, *see* Vasculitis, small-vessel
Angiography
in vasculitis, 171
Angiotensin-converting enzyme inhibitors
use in Raynaud's phenomenon, 161
use in systemic sclerosis, 161
Ankle
disorders, 83–91
examination, 83–88
Ankylosing hyperostosis, *see* Diffuse
idiopathic skeletal hyperostosis
Ankylosing spondylitis, 135–139
Anterior tibial syndrome, *see* Shin splints
Antibiotics, *see also under specific*
antibiotic names
in reactive arthritis, 141
in septic arthritis, 114, 115
Antibodies
anticardiolipin, 21
anticentromere, 21
anti-DNA, 12
anti-dsDNA, 20
anti-Jo-1, 20

Chondromalacia patella, *see*
    Patellofemoral syndrome
Chronic fatigue syndrome, 27, 28, 35
Chronic pain syndromes, 25–38
Cloxactillin, 114
CNS, *see* Central nervous system
Colchicine
    in gout, 105, 109–110
    in polyarteritis nodosa, 171
Colitis, ulcerative
    and spondyloarthropathy, 142
Collars
    in rheumatoid arthritis, 123
    in whiplash, 36
Colles' fracture, *see* Fracture, Colles'
Computed tomography
    in back pain, 153
    in ankylosing spondylitis, 139
Conjunctivitis, *see* Ocular lesions
Corticosteroids
    adverse effects, 198
    in gout, 105, 108–111
    in polymyalgia rheumatica, 46
    in polymyositis/dermatomyositis,
        164–165
    in reflex sympathetic dystrophy, 176
    in rheumatoid arthritis, 204
    in systemic lupus erythematosus, 126,
        128, 131, 132
    in systemic sclerosis, 161
    in vasculitis, 170–174
    local injections, 105, 108–111
Creatine kinase
    in chronic pain syndromes, 34
    in polymyalgia rheumatica, 39
    in polymyositis/dermatomyositis, 14, 40
    causes for elevation of
CREST syndrome, 21, 160, 166
Crystal arthropathy, 102–112
    gout, 103–106, 108–111
    hydroxyapatite deposition disease,
        107–108
    pseudogout, 106–107
Crystal deposition disease
    calcium pyrophosphate, 96, 106–107
    hydroxyapatite, 96, 107–108
    urate, 103–104
Cyclophosphamide
    adverse effects, 169–170
    in polymyositis/dermatomyositis, 165

in rheumatoid arthritis, 203
in systemic lupus erythematosus, 129,
    130
in systemic sclerosis, 161
in vasculitis, 171–173
Cyclosporin
    in polymyositis/dermatomyositis, 165
    in rheumatoid arthritis, 201

Danazol
    in systemic lupus erythematosus, 129,
        130
De Quervain's tendinitis, *see* Tendinitis,
    De Quervain's
Degenerative disc disease, *see* Disc
    degeneration
Dermatomyositis, *see* Polymyositis
Diagnostic criteria, 10–17
Diclofenac, 194
Diffuse idiopathic skeletal hyperostosis,
    95
Diflunisal, 194
Disc degeneration, 95
Disc disease, *see* Disc degeneration
Disc prolapse, 148, 154
Disease-modifying drugs, *see* Slow-acting
    antirheumatic drugs
DISH, *see* Diffuse idiopathic skeletal
    hyperostosis
DMARDs, *see* Slow-acting antirheumatic
    drugs
Drug-induced lupus, 130
DVT, *see* Thrombosis, venous

Effusion, *see* examination of specific
    joints
Elbow
    disorders, 54–58
    examination, 55–56
Enthesitis, 134
Environmental allergy syndrome, *see* The
    Vapours
Erythema
    and arthritis, 77, 103
Erythrocyte sedimentation rate, 18–19
    in chronic pain syndromes, 34
    in giant cell arteritis, 14
    in polymyalgia rheumatica, 14, 39
    in polymyositis/dermatomyositis, 163
    normal values according to age, 19

in systemic lupus erythematosus, 12, 128
Pseudogout, *see* Crystal arthropathy, pseudogout
Psoriatic arthritis, *see* Arthritis, psoriatic
Psychological disorders, *see* Chronic pain syndromes
Psychosis
  corticosteroid induced, 129, 196
  in systemic lupus erythematosus, 12, 129
Pulmonary disease
  in rheumatoid arthritis, 120, 121
  in systemic lupus erythematosus, 12, 127, 128
  in systemic sclerosis, 159
  in vasculitis, 168, 172
  pleural effusion
    in rheumatoid arthritis, 120, 121
    in systemic lupus erythematosus, 127, 128
  pneumonia
    in rheumatoid arthritis, 121
    in systemic lupus erythematosus, 127, 128
  pneumonitis
    drug-induced, 121
    in rheumatoid arthritis, 120, 121
    in systemic lupus erythematosus, 127, 128
Purpura
  in vasculitis, 172
Pyogenic arthritis, *see* Arthritis, septic

Quadriceps exercise, 216

Range of movement, *see* specific regional examination
Raynaud's phenomenon
  in systemic lupus erythematosus, 127, 129
  in systemic sclerosis, 159–161
Reflex algodystrophy, *see* Reflex sympathetic dystrophy
Reflex sympathetic dysfunction, 36
Reflex sympathetic dystrophy, 175–176
  versus chronic pain syndrome, 36
Reiter's syndrome, *see* Arthritis, reactive
Renal biopsy
  in systemic lupus erythematosus, 127

in vasculitis, 168, 199
Renal disease
  drug-induced, 193, 200
  in systemic lupus erythematosus, 12, 127, 128
  in systemic sclerosis, 161
  in vasculitis, 168, 171, 173
Repetitive strain syndrome, 27, 34
Respiratory disease, *see* Pulmonary disease
Retinal lesions, *see* Ocular lesions
Rheumatic fever
  in children, 188
Rheumatoid arthritis, *see* Arthritis, rheumatoid
Rotator cuff tendinitis, *see* Tendinitis, supraspinatus

SAARDs, *see* Slow-acting antirheumatic drugs
Sacroiliitis, *see* Seronegative spondyloarthropathy
Salazopyrin, *see* Sulfasalazine
Salicylates, 194
Salsalate, 194
Scleritis, *see* Ocular lesions
Scleroderma, *see* Systemic sclerosis
Septic arthritis, *see* Arthritis, septic
Serology, *see* specific autoantibody, 18–23
  and diagnostic criteria, 10–12, 23
Seronegative spondyloarthropathy, 13, 133–142
  ankylosing spondylitis, 135–139
  reactive arthritis, 140–141
  psoriatic arthritis, 140–141
  bowel-associated, 142
Shin splints, 91
Shoulder
  disorders, 42–53
  examinations, 43–50
Sicca syndrome, *see* Sjögren's syndrome
Sjögren's syndrome
  in systemic lupus erythematosus, 130
  in systemic sclerosis, 161
  serologic findings, 21
Skeletal scintigraphy, *see* Bone scans
Slow-acting anti-rheumatic drugs, *see also under specific drug name*
Small-vessel vasculitis, *see* Vasculitis, small-vessel

NSAID-induced, *see* NSAIDs, adverse
    effects
oral, *see* Oral lesions
Urethritis, 13, 140
Uric acid levels, 103, 104, 111
Urine abnormalities
    in systemic lupus erythematosus, 12,
        127, 128
    in vasculitis, 168
    drug-induced, 199, 200
Uveitis, *see* Ocular lesions

Vaccination arthritis, *see* Arthritis, post-
    immunization
Valgus
    of ankles, 84
    of hallux, 85
    of knees, 75, 76
Vancomycin
    in septic arthritis, 114
Varus
    of ankles, 84
    of knees, 75, 76
Vasculitis
    and ANCA serology, 22, 173
    classification, 169
    hepatitis B association, 170
    giant cell arteritis, 14, 39, 169, 173
    in Behcet's disease, 169

in rheumatoid arthritis, 120, 121
in search of, 168
in systemic lupus erythematosus,
    126
large vessel, 169, 171
necrotizing, 169
    polyarteritis nodosa, 170
    Wegener's granulomatosus, 172
small vessel, 169, 170
Vertebral fractures *see* Fractures,
    vertebral
Viral arthritis, *see* Arthritis, post-viral
Vitamin D
    in osteoporosis, 180
    levels in bone diseases, 178
Ulcerative colitis, *see* Colitis, ulcerative

Venous thrombosis, *see* Thrombosis,
    venous

Wegener's granulomatosus, *see* Vasculitis,
    necrotizing
Whiplash, 36, 158
Wrist
    disorders, 65
    examination, 63

X-ray findings, *see under specific
    disorders*

ORDERING DETAILS

Main address for orders

BIOS Scientific Publishers Ltd
9 Newtec Place, Magdalen Road,
Oxford OX4 1RE, UK
Tel: +44 1865 726286
Fax: +44 1865 246823

Australia and New Zealand
DA Information Services
648 Whitehorse Road, Mitcham, Victoria 3132, Australia
Tel: (03) 9210 7777
Fax: (03) 9210 7788

India
Viva Books Private Ltd
4325/3 Ansari Road, Daryaganj, New Delhi 110 002, India
Tel: 11 3283121
Fax: 11 3267224

Singapore and South East Asia
(Brunei, Hong Kong, Indonesia, Korea, Malaysia, the Philippines,
Singapore, Taiwan, and Thailand)
Toppan Company (S) PTE Ltd
38 Liu Fang Road, Jurong, Singapore 2262
Tel: (265) 6666
Fax: (261) 7875

USA and Canada
BIOS Scientific Publishers
PO Box 605, Herndon, VA 20172-0605, USA
Tel: (703) 435 7064
Fax: (703) 689 0660

Payment can be made by cheque or credit card (Visa/Mastercard, quoting number
and expiry date). Alternatively, a *pro forma* invoice can be sent.

Prepaid orders must include £2.50/US$5.00 to cover postage and packing
(two or more books sent post free)